Contents

CW00631437

Preface

1.0 General

2.0 Organ failure   29

3.0 Shock   93

4.0 Specific problems   137

Useful values   237

Appendices   247

Index   253

1

Preface

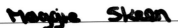

This book is designed to give a concise guide to the management of most acute emergencies. The first part is devoted to the function of and indications for admission to an ITU, monitoring, and basic principles relating to drug therapy.

In all subsequent sections, the text is brief, reinforced by tables for ready reference. The second part is devoted to the management of various aspects of organ failure. The third deals with shock, its pathophysiology and management relating to alterations of fluid balance (including haemorrhagic shock, trauma and sepsis). The fourth section describes management of specific problems—acute disorders secondary to changes in body temperature, metabolic disorders, endocrine crises, disorders of the nervous system, gastro-intestinal emergencies and poisoning.

The purpose of the Pocket Consultant series is to give concise advice, and for this reason discussion is limited. Some of the more important references relating to each section are included.

The book should prove valuable as a rapid therapeutic guide to all doctors working in acute medicine, and for personnel working in acute areas such as Accident and Emergency Departments, ITUs, and operating theatres.

The authors are grateful to Mrs M. Fowler and Mrs J. Snell for their secretarial assistance.

1.0 General

1.1 The function of an ITU, 7

1.2 Indications for admission to an ITU, 7

1.3 Monitoring in an ITU, 7

1.4 Treatment priorities, 8

1.5 Drug therapy in the ITU: General principles, 8

1.6 Tables, 14

1.7 References, 27

1.0 General

1.1 Function / 1.2 Admission / 1.3 Monitoring

1.1 The function of an ITU

An ITU (Intensive Therapy Unit) is a specialist unit providing a facility available to the medical staff for the care of patients who are deemed recoverable but who need continuous supervision and need, or are likely to need, prompt use of specialized techniques by skilled personnel. (BMA Association Planning Unit, 1967.)

In teaching hospitals, the units may be broken up into specialities, e.g. post-cardiotomy care, renal, cardiac—but in the district general hospital the unit is responsible for handling all types of emergency and may have a separate coronary care unit, or this may be a subsection of the general ITU.

1.2 Indications for admission to an ITU

Major indication stated in 1.1. The unit may also be used for specialist techniques where monitoring and resuscitation facilities are readily available, e.g. pericardial tap, lung biopsy, d.c. (direct current) cardioversion, or preparing a sick patient for a major operative procedure.

1.3 Monitoring in an ITU

Objective

Monitoring systems are used to evaluate the physiological derangements present, to observe trends, and to apply appropriate therapy in order to correct any abnormality which, if left, might adversely affect patient prognosis.

Monitoring system types

The systems may be non-invasive, require blood or fluid analysis, or be invasive. The monitoring systems requiring blood or fluid analysis are referred to in the relevant chapters. Non-invasive and invasive systems, their value and limitations, are summarized in Tables 1.1 and 1.2 on pp. 14-19.

1.4 Treatment priorities

The traditional sequence of treatment, namely establishing a diagnosis and then instituting treatment based on the diagnosis, may not be possible because of the critical state of the patient.

Whilst treatment is being established, it is essential to obtain a history, since this may be an important clue to the diagnosis. Frequently, the patient is too ill to give a history, and this must be obtained from the nearest friend or relative.

Treatment should be based on reliable pathophysiological data, 'blind' treatment being only necessary when minutes cannot be spent in waiting for results. Once treatment has been established, the cause for the abnormalities can be sought.

A classic example of this system of patient management is seen in the shocked patient. Treatment is based upon monitoring indices and various blood analyses, and having established the main cause for the shock state (e.g. hypovolaemia) this is treated and the hypovolaemic source then found.

1.5 Drug therapy in the ITU: General principles

The majority of patients in an ITU require drug therapy. Frequently this is multiple, complex, and has to be given intravenously.

Certain basic principles apply:
1 Drug therapy should be kept to the minimum.
2 It is wise, if at all possible, to use drugs of known activity with minimal side-effects.
3 Prescriptions must be precise, written legibly, and revised daily.
4 Drug dosage must be regulated according to individual patient requirements.
5 Drugs given intravenously are best given as a bolus — and should be given into a peripheral vein (multiple injections into a central line increases the incidence of sepsis).
6 It has been suggested by D'Arcy & Griffin (1974) that before any drug is added to any infusion fluid container the following questions should be asked:
   • is it necessary that the drug should be given in this way?

- is the stability of the particular drug in the selected infusion fluid of each drug in the presence of others firmly established?
- if multiple additives are intended, is the stability in the selected infusion fluid of each drug in the presence of the others firmly established?
- will the drug(s) have the intended therapeutic effect if given in high dilution over a period of hours?
- since many drugs decompose slowly in infusion fluids, will the interval between drug addition and use of fluid be kept to a minimum? Also, if the duration of the actual infusion is kept short, will it be compatible with the treatment regimen?

Drugs, when added to an infusion fluid, should be added to normal saline or 1/5 N saline unless the infusion medium is stipulated by the manufacturer. On occasions, the volume advised by the manufacturer for infusion of a drug is excessive in a patient where sodium and volume load is at a premium. Under such circumstances, advice should be sought from the manufacturer.

General pharmacology

This can be divided into *pharmacodynamics* (studies of the biological and therapeutic effects of drugs) and *pharmacokinetics* (studies of the absorption, distribution, metabolism and excretion of drugs).

Three books on pharmacology should be readily available in an ITU:
British National Formulary (1984) (7)
Goodman & Gilman (1982) in *The Pharmacological Basis of Therapeutics*, and
Martindale (1977) in *The Extra Pharmacopoeia*
Readily available senior pharmaceutical advice is also essential.

Pharmacological principles relating to treatment of the critically ill

1 Absorption from the intestinal tract is unpredictable and therefore is rarely used as a therapeutic route.
2 Subcutaneous and intramuscular routes must be avoided when the patient is hypoperfused.

3 Drugs given rectally may, on occasion, be valuable (when the patient is well perfused) giving a prolonged, smooth effect (e.g. rectal dextromoramide for prolonged analgesia).

4 Drugs, when given intravenously, must be given with the administrator being fully aware of the possible hazards.

5 Because of the likelihood of multiple drug therapy being indicated, with some of these drugs being given as an infusion, a full knowledge of adverse drug interactions is essential (Griffin & D'Arcy, 1979).

6 The majority of critically ill patients are suffering from a degree of organ failure; drug metabolism and excretion may therefore be radically affected.

Drug interactions

Drug interactions can occur inside or outside the body. The many possible sites for drug interactions are shown in Fig. 1.1 on p. 11.

Oral drug interactions

Absorption considerably slowed in the presence of ileus; opiates and anticholinergics delay gastric emptying. Salts of divalent or trivalent metals (Ca^{2+} Mg^{2+} Fe^{2+} Al^{3+}) may interact with drugs in the intestine to produce insoluble and non-absorbable complexes. Intestinal flow may be suppressed due to antibiotic therapy—this reduces the manufacture of vitamin K and may increase the anticoagulant effect of anticoagulant therapy.

Drug interactions due to enzyme induction

Many interactions are due to drug-metabolizing enzymes which are sited predominantly in the liver and may be affected by preceding administration of other drugs. These enzymes may be induced and hence reduce activity (Table 1.1), or may be inhibited and hence increase subsequent drug activity. The latter is rarely of relevance during intensive therapy except that chloramphenicol may inhibit enzymes responsible for metabolizing warfarin.

A patient who has taken a tricyclic overdose may potentiate the effect of catecholamines by inhibition of their uptake; they are known to increase the lethality of digoxin especially in the presence of stress.

1.5 Drug therapy in the ITU

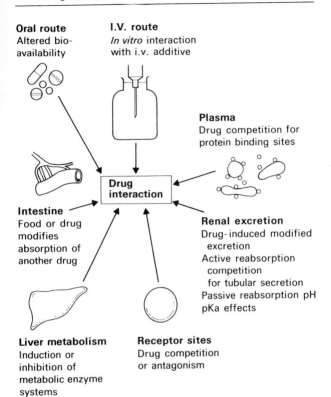

Oral route
Altered bio-
availability

I.V. route
In vitro interaction
with i.v. additive

Plasma
Drug competition for
protein binding sites

Drug interaction

Intestine
Food or drug
modifies
absorption of
another drug

Renal excretion
Drug-induced modified
 excretion
Active reabsorption
 competition
 for tubular secretion
Passive reabsorption pH
pKa effects

Liver metabolism
Induction or
inhibition of
metabolic enzyme
systems

Receptor sites
Drug competition
or antagonism

Fig. 1.1. Sites of drug interactions.

Drug interactions at plasma and receptor-binding sites

Important changes in drug distribution can arise from competition
between drugs for protein-binding sites in plasma or tissues.

Drug interactions in excretory mechanisms

Passive reabsorption. A non-protein-bound drug is filtered at the
glomerulus and is progressively concentrated as water is reabsorbed during its passage down the nephron. A concentration
gradient is established and, if the drug is lipid-soluble and able to
permeate the tubular epithelium, it will be passively reabsorbed

back into the systemic circulation. Many drugs are weak electrolytes, and passive reabsorption can only occur in the non-ionized lipid soluble form; the degree of ionization is determined by the pH of the renal environment and therefore changes in tubular fluid pH must influence excretion of the drug.

Thus, acid urine favours the ionization of alkaline drugs (and vice versa) so that reabsorption is reduced and renal excretion is increased. These effects are only of clinical significance when the pKa (dissociation constant) of the drug is 7.5-10.5 for bases and 3.0-7.5 for acids. The effect of urinary pH on the pKa of a drug is used in the treatment of drug overdose, (a detailed list of pKa's is available in Martindale, 1977) and may also prolong or decrease the effect of drug therapy should urinary pH be altered by (for example) the infusion of sodium bicarbonate.

Other factors in drug interactions

Drugs affecting liver or renal blood flow may affect drug activity. The rate of metabolism or elimination of a drug may also be affected by the shock state leading to renal and hepatic hypoperfusion. Drug interactions of particular relevance during the treatment of the critically ill are summarized in Table 1.3.

Drug metabolism

Patients who have suffered a period of hypotension are likely to have sustained a degree of liver and/or renal hypoperfusion — this may lead to delayed metabolism and/or decreased excretion respectively. Drugs which may have a prolonged activity as a result of impaired function of these organs are summarized in Tables 1.4 and 1.5.

Benzodiazepines are used extensively in the ITU, and the choice depends upon the therapeutic requirements, the likely duration of their use, and hepatic function (see Tables 1.5-1.6). The benzodiazepines with acute metabolites should be avoided when prolonged use is anticipated. Benzodiazepines should be used with caution in patients with hepatocellular dysfunction; a short-acting agent with no active metabolites should be selected and used in low dosage, the dose being titrated according to the therapeutic response (Table 1.6).

1.0 General

1.5 Drug therapy in the ITU

Therapeutic efficacy

In certain instances, blood level monitoring is important in order to ensure therapeutic efficacy. It is particularly important where high levels may produce dangerous side-effects, or where the drug is ineffective below a certain level.

Therapeutic blood levels of particular importance in the ITU (including patients with poisoning) are summarized in Table 1.7.

Table 1.1. Non-invasive monitoring systems

System	Value	Limitations

Pulse rate	One of the best indicators of 'stress'
	Inc. early indicator of hypovolaemia, sepsis
	Inc. in carbondiozide retention, hypoxia (bradycardia in profound hypoxia) and a metabolic acidosis
	Inappropriate bradycardia in the presence of stress
	may be due to: drugs
	          myocardial depression
	          cardiac conduction defects
		Pulse rate may be radically affected by drugs:
		    beta blockers
		    atropine
		    neostigmine
		    heminevrin
		    certain hypotensives
		    epidural blockade
		with local anaesthetic agents:
		    certain inhalational anaesthetics

ECG trace	Detection of cardiac dysrhythmias and conduction defects
	Detection of changes in ionic balance, in particular potassium, calcium and magnesium.
	Drug toxicity, e.g.
	    tricyclics
	    digitalis
	    phenothiazines
		Essential that ECG leads are placed correctly and maintained in the same position between observations.
		Electrical interference

Blood pressure	Adequate systolic pressure essential for organ perfusion	Cuff technique unreliable at low levels

	High pulse pressure with normal skin temperature may be evidence of diminished SVR (systemic vascular resistance)	Doppler non-invasive technique more reliable
	High pulse pressure classic in thyrotoxicosis	SP <70 mmHg — intra-arterial line for reliable levels
	Low SP (systolic pressure) clinically present in all shock states, the exceptions being where the SP falls below normal for that patient, e.g. preceding hypertension, eclampsia	SP not a reliable indicator of CO
	Pulse pressure a reasonable indicator of CO (cardiac output)	Pulse pressure not a reliable indicator of CO once SP <90 mmHg

Temperature
Core temperature
(central body temperature)
	High core temperature may indicate sepsis
	Rapidly rising core temperature, in particular in a child, may precede convulsions
	High temperature in the absence of sepsis may indicate:
	    dehydration
	    thyrotoxicosis
	    an autoimmune disorder
	    salicylate intoxication
	Low core temperature may be a manifestation of:
	    hypothyroidism, panhypopituitrism
	    exposure
	    drugs—phenothiazines
		Measurement by rectal probe may be unreliable and easily becomes displaced. Oesophageal readings or core temperature readings more reliable

continued

Table 1.1—*continued*

Skin temperature	Low skin temperature evidence of poor perfusion. Useful following vascular surgery and as an indicator of skin perfusion in shock	Unreliable as an indicator of trends in shock in the presence of peripheral vascular disease
Skin/core temperature differential	High level classic of severe shock, valuable as a sequential guide to trends in skin perfusion	
Respiratory rate	Raised in hypoxia, increased oxygen demands resp. stimulation, e.g. salicylates decreased in CNS (central nervous system) depression due to: CO$_2$ narcosis drugs brain pathology	Resp. rate may be depressed due to drugs, e.g. opiates
Tidal volume	Dec. due to: CNS pathology neuromuscular disease pulmonary pathology drugs	Difficult to measure with accuracy unless E-T (endotracheal) tube or tracheostomy present

1.6   Tables

	Particularly valuable during patient weaning from a ventilator, observation of trends, in neuro-muscular disease (Guillain-Barré syndrome, myasthenia gravis) and as an indicator of severe CNS depression due to drug intoxication	Patient co-operation and correct technique essential
Peak flow	Valuable in observation of trends in the severe asthmatic	
FEV_1 (forced expiratory volume over 1 sec)	Rarely performed in an ITU setting	

Table 1.2. Invasive monitoring systems

System	Value	Limitations/dangers
Arterial blood pressure	Accurate measurement of SP and DP (diastolic pressure) Measurement of severe hypotension and hypertension Valuable in order to recognize trends, e.g. during hypotensive therapy or treatment of shock. Easy access for blood sampling	Standardized electric equipment required. Ischaemic gangrene if no cross circulation present Haemorrhage
Right atrial pressure	Estimate of inflow volume to the right heart. Accurate reflector of hypovolaemia Normal values may be present in the presence of hypovolaemia and left-sided failure. Essential to assess right-sided tolerance based on the fluid challenge (p. 104)	Inaccurate reflector of LV (left ventricular) function; inappropriate use may lead to fluid overload Level may be raised by increased intra-thoracic pressure, increased pulmonary vascular resistance or pulmonary hypotension in the presence of a low or normal PCWP (pulmonary capillary wedge pressure) Essential that line is monitored correctly. Numerous dangers related to insertion; subsequent dangers include air embolism and sepsis

1.6 Tables

Pulmonary capillary wedge pressure (PCWP)	Reflector of LAP (left atrial pressure) and hence an indicator of LV performance Valuable in shock states where impairment of LV function is suspected Valuable in situations where the RAP (right atrial pressure) is high and yet hypovolaemia is suspected	Unreliable readings are more dangerous than no readings at all Back-up facilities are considerable. Insertion should be performed by an experienced clinician and maintenance by skilled personnel
Cardiac output (CO) Cardiac index (CI) (CO/BSA l^{-1} min^{-1} m^{-2})	In conjunction with the PCWP in order to optimize volume replacement Optimization of ventilation/perfusion in the patient with serious pulmonary pathology Evaluation of drug response in serious non-hypovolaemic shock states Evaluation of drug response in severe hypotension	Level may be artificially raised during ventilation with high airway pressures or during the application of PEEP (positive end expiratory pressure) Numerous dangers related to insertion; subsequent dangers include: sepsis air embolism pulmonary haemorrhage
Systemic vascular resistance (SVR)	Indicator of the state of the peripheral vascular system and may be used in conjunction with the CO and PCWP to decide upon the most appropriate drug to use in conditions of shock Response to drug therapy—in shock and hypotensive therapy	A derived value from SVR (mmHg l^{-1} min.M^{-2}) $$\frac{MAP - RAP\ (mmHg)^*}{CI}$$

*MAP, mean atrial pressure

Table 1.3. Some drug interactions due to enzyme induction of particular relevance during management of the critically ill

Enzyme inducer	Drug activity reduced by enhanced metabolism
Alcohol	Phenobarbitone Phenytoin Warfarin
Barbiturates	Corticosteroids Coumarin anticoagulants Phenytoin
Phenytoin	Corticosteroids
Long-term antibiotic therapy Benzpyrene (component of tobacco smoke)	Antibiotics Pentazocine Benzodiazepines

Table 1.4. Drugs commonly used in the ITU which should be avoided or used with caution in renal failure

Drug	Creatinine clearance ml/min below which dosage must be reduced*	Dosage recommendation comments
GI (gastro-intestinal) tract		
Cimetidine	10-20	600 mg daily
Magnesium trisilicate	< 10	Avoid
Cardiovascular drugs		
Diazoxide	< 10	75-150 mg i.v.
Hydralazine	< 10	Start small dose
Beta-blockers	< 10	See table on p. 70
Digoxin	20-50	250 μg daily
Anti-arrhythmics		
Mexilitine	< 20	Reduce dosage

1.0 General

1.6 Tables

Disopyramide	20-50	100 mg every 8 h
	10-20	100 mg every 12 h
	< 10	100 mg every 24 h
Procainamide	< 50	Avoid or reduce dosage
Tocainide	< 50	Reduce dosage
Diuretics		
Ethacrynic acid	< 10	Avoid ototoxic
Frusemide	< 20	May need high doses; deafness with rapid infusion
Central nervous system (CNS)		
Phenobarbitone	< 10	Avoid
Aspirin	< 10	Avoid
Pethidine	< 10	Avoid
Haloperidol	< 20	Reduce dosage
Droperidol	< 20	Reduce dosage
Infections		
Aminoglycosides	< 50	Reduce dosage, regulating according to blood levels Ototoxic Nephrotoxic
Amphotericin	< 50	Use only if essential Nephrotoxic
Cephalosporins		
Cephaloridine	< 50	Avoid
Others	< 50	Reduce dosage
Chloramphenicol	< 10	Avoid unless no alternative
Cycloserine	< 50	Avoid
Ethambutol	< 50	Reduce dosage Optic nerve damage
Isoniazid	< 10	Max. 200 mg daily Peripheral neuropathy
Metronidazole	< 20	Reduce dosage

continued

Table 1.4 — *continued*

Penicillins			
Amoxycillin	< 10		Reduce dosage
Ampicillin	< 10		Max. 250 mg every 8 h
Benzyl penicillin	< 10		Max. 6 g daily
Carbenicillin	< 50		Use alternative
Sulphonamides	< 10		Avoid
Tetracyclines except Doxycycline Minocycline	< 50		Avoid
Bronchodilators			
Aminophylline	< 20		Reduce dosage

*Appropriate relationship between creatinine clearance and serum creatinine as follows:

Creatinine clearance (ml/min)	Serum creatinine (μmol/l)
25-50	150-300 (approx.)
10-20	300-700 (approx.)
< 10	> 700 (approx.)

Table 1.5. Drugs commonly used in the ITU which are inactivated by hepatic metabolism

Anti-arrhythmics
Lignocaine
Tocainade
Procainamide
Mexilitine
Quinidine
Verapamil

Antibiotics
Chloramphenicol
Clindamycin
Isoniazid
Rifampicin

Anticonvulsants
Phenobarbitone
Phenytoin
Valproic acid

Bronchodilators
Aminophylline

Antihypertensives
Majority of beta blockers
Hydralazine
Prazosin

Narcotic analgesics
Opiates
Pentazocine
Pethidine
Phenoperidine
Fentanyl

Phenothiazines
Chlorpromazine

Sedatives
Chlordiazepoxide
Certain benzodiazepines
(see table on p. 23)

Steroids

Table 1.6. Classification of benzodiazepines

Short-acting	Active metabolites
Lorazepam	No
Oxazepam	No
Temazepam	No
Triazolam	Yes
Long-acting	
Diazepam	Yes
Chlordiazepoxide	Yes
Clorazepate	Yes
Medazepam	Yes
Clobazam	Yes
Ketazolam	Yes
Nitrazepam	No
Flurazepam	Yes
Clonazepam	No

Table 1.7. Therapeutic and toxic blood levels of drugs used and encountered in the ITU

	Therapeutic concentration (mg/l)	Toxic concentration (mg/l)	Lethal or potentially lethal concentration (mg/l)
Aminophylline	10-20	20	—
Amitriptyline	50-200 μg/l	400 μg/l	10-20
Barbiturates			
short acting	1	7	10
intermediate	1-5	10-30	30
phenobarbitone	15	40-70	80-150
Bromide	50	0.5-1.5 g/l	2 g/l
Carbon monoxide	1% saturation of Hb	15-35% saturation of Hb	50% saturation of Hb
Chlordiazepoxide	1.0-2.0	6	20
Desipramine	0.59-1.4	—	—
Dextropropoxyphane	50-200 μg/l	—	—
Diazepam	0.5-2.5	5-20	50

Disopyramide	2.8-4.1 µg/l	5.5 µg/l	—
Digoxin	1-2 µg/l	2-9 µg/l	—
Gentamicin peak level 1 h after i.m. injection	4-8 µg/l	10 µg/ml	
Glutethimide	1-5	10-30	30-100
Imipramine	0.1-0.3	0.7	2
Iron		6 (serum)	
Lead	0.05-1.3	1.3	—
Lignocaine	2-4	6	—
Lithium	0.8-1.2 mmol/l	1.5 mmol/l	4 mmol/l
Meprobamate	10	100	200
Methanol	—	200	890
Mexilitine	0.6-2.5	—	—
Morphine	0.1	—	0.5-4
Nortriptyline	50-200 µg/l	400 µg/l	10-20
Paracetamol	5-25	30	250 at 4 h 50 at 12 h

continued

Table 1.7—*continued*

Pentazocine	0.1-1	2-5	10-20
Pethidine	600-650 μg/l	5	30
Phenytoin	8-20	30	100
Primidone	10	50-80	100
Prochlorperazine	—	1	—
Promazine	—	1	—
Propranolol	0.025-0.1	—	8-12
Salicylate (methyl salicylic acid)	100-350	350-400	500
Theophylline	10-20	20	—
Tricyclics	50-200 μg/l	400 μg/l	10-20

1.7 References

British National Formulary (1984) (7) British Medical Association and the Pharmaceutical Society of Great Britain.

D'Arcy P.F. & Griffin J.P. (1974) Drug interactions, 2: By mixing drugs before administration. *Prescribers' J.* **14**, 38-40.

Goodman L.S. & Gilman A. (1982) - In *The Pharmacological Basis of Therapeutics.* (Ed. by A.G. Gilman, L.S. Goodman & A. Gilman), 6th ed. Macmillan Inc., New York.

Griffin J.P. & D'Arcy P.F. (1979) *A Manual of Adverse Drug Interactions*, 2nd ed. J. Wright & Sons Ltd, Bristol.

Martindale (1977) In *The Extra Pharmacopoeia* (Ed. by A. Wade), 27th ed. Pharmaceutical Press, London.

1.0 General

Notes
_____

2.0 Organ failure

2.1 Cardiac disorders, 31
Cardiac arrest
Cardiac arrhythmias
Cardiac failure
Acute hypertensive crisis

2.2 Respiratory failure, 40 (C.S. Waldmann)
Introduction
General management
Adult respiratory distress syndrome (ARDS)
Fat embolism syndrome
Near drowning
Pulmonary aspiration syndrome
Pulmonary embolism
Asthma
Chest injuries

2.3 Hepatic failure, 55
Introduction
Clinical features
Treatment

2.4 Management of renal failure, 60
Introduction
Treatment of pre-renal failure
Treatment of post-renal failure
Management of acute renal failure

2.5 Tables, 67

2.6 References, 90

2.0 Organ failure

2.1 Cardiac disorders

Cardiac arrest

Definition
Sudden—often unexpected—cessation of effective heart action
with subsequent inadequate brain perfusion.

Diagnosis
Loss of mentation associated with absent carotid or femoral
pulses. Time should not be wasted in auscultation.

Treatment
Summarized in Table 2.1

Comments
It is essential that the patient is on a firm surface. External cardiac
massage is performed by kneeling beside the patient and placing
the base of the hand over the lower sternum; the second hand
is placed over the first in order to maintain the correct position.
The lower part of the sternum is depressed firmly to a depth of
2-4 cm, and the sternum is allowed to rebound by release of the
pressure. The rate should be approximately 60/min. (In a child
one hand is used and in an infant two fingers will suffice.) A
pause is made every four to six compressions to allow lung
inflation. Lung inflation can be continued by mouth-to-nose or
mouth-to-mouth respiration; or with the aid of a resuscitator such
as an Ambu bag face mask and an oropharyngeal airway; a
Brooke airway, or a rebreathing bag with face mask and com-
pressed oxygen. With efficient external cardiac massage and
mouth-to-nose, or mouth-to-mouth resuscitation, adequate
cerebral oxygenation can be maintained for at least 1 h. Stopping
these procedures for even a few seconds may lead to irreparable
cerebral damage. An ECG trace can be obtained quickly by using
pre-gelled disposable electrodes placed under the patient's back.
When an ECG trace cannot be obtained within minutes, blind
d.c. (direct current) shock should be performed. Intracardiac
adrenaline should be used in asystole and in the presence of small
magnitude ventricular fibrillation. The injection is performed using
a fine lumbar puncture needle inserted in the fourth or fifth intercostal space 2-3 inches from the sternum. Successful resuscitation following a period of asystole is rare, and depends upon
the onset of VF (ventricular fibrillation) or the exceptional case
who responds to cardiac pacing.

2.0 Organ failure

2.1 Cardiac disorders

If an ECG trace cannot be obtained quickly, d.c. defibrillation should be performed blind. Points to remember are:

1 Electrode jelly is preferable to KY jelly; place one paddle below the right clavicle and the other over the apex. Do not allow the jelly to run across the chest between the electrodes. During defibrillation the operator must not stand in a puddle of saline or blood and all other personnel must stand away from the bed. At each attempt the electrodes must be smeared with fresh jelly.
2 The d.c. shock should be started at 50 joules, increasing by 50-100 joules on each attempt to 400 joules.
3 Should d.c. shock fail after four attempts, give 100 mg lignocaine intravenously followed by a further shock. In the event of failure to cardiovert on the above regime, check acid base state, PaO_2 (arterial oxygen pressure) and serum potassium and correct any abnormality. Other anti-arrhythmics which may be tried with failed cardioversion include phenytoin sodium, tocainide, procainamide, mexilitine, disopyramide and amiodarone. Drugs which may be considered occasionally include practolol (see p. 70) and bretylium.
4 The use of multiple antidysrhythmiacs must be avoided since asystole or a serious bradyarrhythmia may occur during or following d.c. shock.
5 Once the patient has cardioverted maintain a lignocaine infusion of 1-4 mg/min following a loading dose of 60-120 mg. (Lignocaine in concentration >2 mg/min may be complicated by convulsions.)

Asystole

The prognosis is very poor and most commonly occurs following a prolonged period of VF and/or hypoxia. Attempt to produce VF by intracardiac adrenaline coupled with external cardiac massage. Defibrillate if VF occurs.

Asystole may be due to the following:
• rapid changes in serum potassium
• pulmonary embolism
• hypoxia secondary to pulmonary atelectasis, extreme bronchospasm, bilateral or unilateral pneumothorax

When a rapid fall in serum potassium is likely, potassium chloride 20 mmol in 100 ml 1/5 N saline should be infused over 10 min. In

2.0 Organ failure

2.1 Cardiac disorders

pulmonary embolism, ECM (external cardiac massage) may push the clot peripherally and circulation be restored (see p. 48)

Factors precipitating ventricular fibrillation, which must be excluded, include the factors which may produce asystole, serious electrolyte or acid base balance (including alterations of magnesium and calcium) or drug intoxication (including tricyclic antidepressants, digoxin).

Supportive treatment
Should the arrest have been prolonged (>2 min) the presentation asystole, or spontaneous ventilation not return within 3 min of successful cardioversion, the patient should be electively ventilated. Fixed dilated pupils may persist for several hours post resuscitation with subsequent recovery. It should be assumed that a prolonged arrest may be complicated by cerebral oedema — the patient should be ventilated for at least 24 h maintaining a PaO_2 of 10 kPa (75 mmHg) or greater, and a $PaCO_2$ around 3.7 kPa (28 mmHg).

Check Se K and if >4.5 mmol/l give dexamethasone 4 mg i.v. and mannitol 20% 2 g/kg over 10 min. Mannitol must not be given if renal failure is suspected or RAP (right atrial pressure) >5 cm H_2O.

RAP monitoring is essential and in the presence of an adequate BP (blood pressure), SP (systolic pressure) (90 mmHg or greater) and urine output >40 ml/h it should be kept low (1-5 cm H_2O). Where there is doubt PCWP (pulmonary capillary wedge pressure) monitoring may be considered, keeping in mind that post-arrest passage of a catheter through the tricuspid valve may precipitate a dangerous dysrhythmia.

Post-arrest management (summarized in Table 2.2)
A sustained low BP and poor urine output is an indication for inotrope therapy. Dopamine is the drug of first choice, but should peripheral vasoconstriction be severe or peripheral vasoconstriction develop during therapy, dobutamine should be considered. In the presence of poor peripheral perfusion do not go above 3 μg/kg/min of dopamine before adding dobutamine (see p. 77 and 78).

Pulse rate <60/min — consider cardiac pacing. It is preferable not to use isoprenaline in these circumstances because of the increased metabolic demands with its use.

2.0 Organ failure

2.1 Cardiac disorders

A severe metabolic acidosis (pH < 7.2), a metabolic alkalosis (pH > 7.5) and hypoxia, produce a compensatory increase in cardiac output and should therefore be corrected. Hypovolaemia must be corrected. When there is doubt about the left ventricular pressures, PCWP monitoring should be instituted if at all possible (p. 19)

Any evidence of pulmonary aspiration, atelectasis, pulmonary oedema, is an indication to continue ventilation. Ventilation must be adjusted in order to optimize cardiac output. PEEP (positive end expiratory pressure) should be avoided since it commonly reduces cardiac output when cardiac function is compromised.

In order to achieve sedation, drugs producing pupillary changes should be avoided. Excessive doses of diazepam should not be used because of the prolonged sedative effect related to its metabolites. Where repeated assessment of the cerebral state is necessary use i.v. heminevrin (observe volume) or i.v. etomidate and fentanyl (this may lower the BP).

Ventilated patients not requiring repeated neurological assessment are generally sedated for 24 h and then allowed to gently 'lighten' and, provided PaO_2 is greater than 9.3 kPa (70 mmHg) on an FiO_2 of 0.35 or less and there is no other contraindication to extubation (e.g. crushed chest injury), the patient is extubated once he/she is able to ventilate spontaneously via the endotracheal tube.

With continued use of dexamethasone for cerebral oedema, give adequate K replacement.

Hyperventilation is used in order to decrease cerebral oedema which inevitably arises after a prolonged arrest; ventilation should be adjusted in order to obtain a normal $PaCO_2$ before taking the patient off the ventilator.

Cardiac arrhythmias

Abnormalities in cardiac rhythm occur most commonly in ischaemic heart disease (IHD) but may also be seen in the critically ill, particularly the elderly.

Factors which may contribute to, or precipitate a dysrhythmia, are enumerated in Table 2.3.

2.0 Organ failure

2.1 Cardiac disorders

Drugs most commonly used in the ITU for treatment of dysrhythmias are summarized in Table 2.4.

Important points are:
• exclude any precipitating factor and treat if possible
• is the arrhythmia serious or potentially dangerous?
• has the arrhythmia produced a serious fall in cardiac output?

An abnormal rhythm may be present which will revert spontaneously on eliminating the precipitating factor, or which is not affecting cardiac output and is not potentially serious — under these conditions it is wise to observe and not to treat.

Supraventricular tachycardia (SVT)
The nature of the dysrhythmia can generally be elicited by the ECG. Where the interpretation is difficult, senior advice should be obtained. Diagnosis may be assisted by looking at the atrial rate and A-V (atrial-ventricular) conduction on the ECG (Table 2.5) and observing the response to cardiac massage on the oscilloscope trace.

Treatment of SVT (summarized in Table 2.6). Any SVT may be complicated by the sick sinus syndrome, the WPW (Wolff-Parkinson-White) syndrome or digitalis toxicity — the management of these problems is described on pp. 36 and 169.

Paroxysmal SVT. Carotid sinus massage may be helpful in making the diagnosis and in certain cases may arrest the dysrhythmia.

Digoxin is useful when control is required within 4-6 h but should not be used where toxicity is suspected, where the Se K is low, and should be used with caution in the presence of renal failure. The major factors affecting digoxin therapeutic efficacy are listed in Table 2.7. In the critically ill many factors may have precipitated the dysrhythmia and affect digoxin sensitivity; it is therefore wise to give three doses of 0.5 mg digoxin 3-4 h apart and then to review the dosage. In many instances the rhythm will have changed to sinus and digoxin can be discontinued.

In spite of β-blockade being recommended for paroxysmal SVT, the author prefers to avoid it because of the myocardial suppressant effect and the danger of either inducing bronchospasm or exacerbating existing spasm. Many β-blockers also have the disadvantage that they induce a bradycardia, thereby suppressing the normal cardiac response to stress, namely a tachycardia with an increase in CO (cardiac output).

Verapamil may be particularly valuable in the younger age group. In the elderly, where the haemodynamic state is compromised or where either digoxin or a negative inotrope is inadvisable, synchronized d.c. shock is the most suitable treatment. Cardioversion may be possible with low shock levels; it is preferable to start at 25 joules, gradually increasing to 400 joules until cardioversion occurs. Should cardioversion not have occurred at 200 joules, any factor which may perpetuate the tachycardia should be treated if at all possible.

Following cardioversion, verapamil or digoxin should be used for 24 h in the hope of preventing recurrence.

Atrial fibrillation (AF). Where AF is thought to be of recent onset, the patient young and the precipitating factors resolved, cardioversion is the treatment of choice. Where the patient is elderly and the underlying cause still present, rapid digitalization is most suitable. Frequently, digitalization will lead to cardioversion within 24 h. The dosage of digoxin required for maintenance (should AF continue) must be individually tailored, taking note of factors which may affect therapeutic efficacy (see Table 2.6).

Paroxysmal SVT or AF with the WPW syndrome. Under such circumstances (if the haemodynamic state is compromised) cardioversion should be performed followed by maintenance disopyramide. Quinidine or amiodarone are alternative maintenance drugs. In less acute conditions the SVT may be controlled by i.v. disopyramide. Digoxin *must be* avoided.

Paroxysmal SVT or AF complicated by the sick sinus syndrome. It is wise to avoid carotid sinus massage, verapamil and/or β-blockade since a dangerous bradyarrhythmia may develop. Direct current (d.c.) cardioversion is probably the safest treatment for immediate relief but in rare instances, because of the onset of a bradyarrhythmia, cardiac pacing may be necessary.

Following cardioversion, amiodarone or disopyramide should be considered as a prophylactic.

Ventricular tachyarrhythmia (VT) (summarized in Table 2.8) *Decelerated idioventricular rhythm.* This rarely requires treatment; the higher rates, however, (110-120/min) are closely related to VT.

2.0 Organ failure

2.1 Cardiac disorders

Ventricular tachycardia (VT). This is a tachycardia associated with a broad QRS complex at a rate of 120-240 beats/min. Should the attack be prolonged haemodynamic performance is generally impaired.

Torsade de pointes is a form of VT with changes in direction of the QRS axis over runs of 5-20 beats. Cardioversion has only a temporary effect; i.v. isoprenaline should be used to shorten repolarization time, followed by cardiac pacing.

In torsade de pointes certain precipitating factors must be treated: hypokalaemia; hypomagnesaemia; anti-arrhythmic or psycho-tropic drugs. VT may be precipitated post infarction or by a bradycardia—this should be treated with atropine. Should there be haemodynamic impairment, d.c. shock is the treatment of choice, followed by a lignocaine infusion.

In the ITU it is probably wise to cardiovert—as opposed to using drugs—but where the patient's tolerance is good and there are contraindications to anaesthesia (e.g. recent heavy meal), then the following drugs may be used intravenously (see Table 2.4): lignocaine; tocainide; mexiletine; procainamide; phenytoin; amiodarone.

Bradycardia. Sinus bradycardia is common post myocardial infarc-tion and generally responds to atropine. Atropine should be tried in any bradyarrhythmia associated with syncope, hypotension, cardiac failure or ventricular ectopic rhythm. Under the above circumstances, *cardiac pacing* is indicated should atropine fail.

Other indications for cardiac pacing include:
- Stokes-Adams attacks
- low output states associated with a bradycardia unresponsive to atropine (isoprenaline may be used as a temporary measure)
- inferior infarction if the heart rate <60/min
- if anterior infarction indications controversial—generally pace in the presence of CHB, RBBB/PFB and alternating RBBB/LBBB
- refractory tachycardias
- pre-operatively in the critically ill; pacing is essential in patients asymptomatic with CHB
- bradycardia due to drug overdose (e.g. digoxin, β-blockers)
- carotid sinus syncope
- failed permanent pacemaker

Method of insertion of a temporary pacemaker is described by Pitcher (1982).

2.0 Organ failure

2.1 Cardiac disorders

Cardiac failure

Left ventricular failure (LVF)
LVF in the absence of a serious dysrhythmia, hypertension or severe PVR1. Nurse in the upright position, give sedation with opiates, intravenous diuretics and oxygen via face mask (Table 2.9).

LVF in the presence of serious dysrhythmia. Treat as above but also correct dysrhythmia, preferably by d.c. cardioversion followed by appropriate antidysrhythmic (pp. 34-37). Ensure that is no cardiac cause for the dysrhythmia.

LVF in the presence of cardiogenic shock. Sedation, i.v. diuretics and oxygen are used and further therapy depends upon the haemodynamic problems present. The haemodynamic state should be assessed by means of a Swan-Ganz catheter and measurements of RAP and PCWP; sequential cardiac output measurements (thermodilution technique) are also desirable. SVR can be calculated (p. 19).

Drugs to be considered are inotropes and vasodilators (Table 2.9) and provided haemodynamic monitoring is available, a combination may be necessary.

Isoprenaline should be avoided when there has been a recent ischaemic episode and dopamine should be avoided when there is a high SVR. Once the BP SP has been raised above 80 mmHg SP with an inotrope, a vasodilator should be considered. Isosorbide dinitrate is preferable when there has been recent ischaemia but does little for SVR. Where the SVR is high, the condition potentially rapidly reversible (<24 h) and myocardial ischaemia is present, nitroprusside is the drug of choice. Hydrallazine and isosorbide dinitrate in combination is particularly valuable when LVF is present coupled with a raised SVR and myocardial ischaemia and where the condition is likely to be protracted.

It is important to exclude any factor(s) which are correctable surgically, e.g. valvular disease, congenital heart disease, acute ventricular septal defect (VSD) or LV aneurysm secondary to IHD. Where there is a surgically correctable lesion, it is essential to consult the nearest cardiothoracic unit. Under such circumstances pre-operative balloon counterpulsation may be considered (Yacoub, 1978).

2.0 Organ failure

2.1 Cardiac disorders

Cardiogenic shock in the absence of LVF. Should a dysrhythmia be present this must be corrected and any non-cardiac cause for the dysrhythmia excluded.

Where the PCWP is low, careful volume loading with plasma protein fraction (PPF) should be undertaken until PCWP is 8 mmHg (in the midthoracic position with a normal colloid osmotic pressure (COP)).

In the presence of a normal PCWP an inotrope should be used, the inotrope of choice depending upon the haemodynamic state. A high SVR is an indication for caution in using dopamine because of the danger of the α-adrenergic effect in high doses, and dobutamine or isoprenaline may be considered. Isoprenaline should be avoided when there has been recent myocardial ischaemia but it is valuable in low dosage where there is a bradycardia (Table 2.9).

The dosage of any inotrope should be started at the minimum and slowly increased until SP is 80 mmHg or more and peripheral perfusion has improved.

A refractory acidosis coupled with an increased SVR, hypotension and oliguria/anuria in spite of inotrope therapy are bad prognostic features.

Acute hypertensive crises

Hypertension in general should be taken seriously when the DP (diastolic pressure) is greater than 110 mmHg and the SP greater than 170 mmHg. Under certain conditions lower figures should be treated:
• post operative—following major surgery
• postoperative vascular surgery (e.g. aortic aneurysm repair)
• pre-eclampsia/eclampsia
• preceding history of cerebral haemorrhage
• presence of a recent cerebral catastrophe (e.g. subarachnoid haemorrhage, aortic dissection)
• presence of extreme swings in BP (e.g. phaeochromocytoma, amine oxidase inhibitor associated hypertension due to dietary indiscretion or drug potentiation)

Treatment
Each patient has to be treated on individual grounds and the type

of drug used depends upon the clinical history, the acuteness of onset and the rate at which it is desirable to lower BP.

In general
The BP should be lowered over a period of hours to a DP around 100 mmHg the exception being the above where it may be desirable to lower the SP to less than 150 mmHg and DP to less than 90 mmHg within 30 min. The drug selected should be preferably titrated intravenously with intra-arterial monitoring control.

In postoperative cases and where circulating volume is uncertain (e.g. phaeochromocytoma, pre-eclampsia), a RAP line is essential since dangerous and sudden hypotension may occur with the use of a peripheral vasodilator.

The agents which have proved must useful are enumerated in Table 2.10 and the procedure for lowering BP is given in Table 2.11.

2.2 Respiratory failure (by C.S. Waldmann)

Introduction

Respiratory failure is defined as inability to maintain $PaO_2 > 8$ kPa(60 mmHg) and $PaCO_2 < 6.7$ kPa(50 mmHg) whilst breathing air at sea-level. The levels of blood gases at which a diagnosis of respiratory failure is made are somewhat arbitrary. It is wise to make an age allowance for the normal PaO_2 thus:

$$PaO_2 = (104 - \underline{Age})/7.5 \text{ kPa (Mellemgraad, 1966)}$$
$$4$$

Causes
- type 1 — hypoxaemia without CO_2 retention in which there is normal or increased alveolar ventilation
- type II — hypoxaemia with CO_2 retention in which ventilation is reduced
- diagnosis
- blood gases

N.B. If analysis cannot be immediately performed keep the sample on ice. Investigation of the cause of respiratory failure should be undertaken if the cause is not obvious. See Tables 2.12 and 2.13.

2.0 Organ failure

2.2 Respiratory failure

General management

In severe chronic pulmonary diseases, heroic measures are best withheld unless there is an acute and potentially reversible component to their condition. In these cases you should ask the advice of your consultant.

Physiotherapy and postural drainage
Summarized in Table 2.14.

Antibiotics
These should be withheld until sputum and blood cultures are taken. Their use in the absence of definite evidence of infection remains controversial.

Fluid balance
This should be carefully controlled. Colloid osmotic pressure (COP) should be measured and maintained. Patients with low COP have a poor prognosis. At low albumin levels COP correlates well with total plasma protein concentration but not with albumin concentration. Prevention of pulmonary oedema in these patients is imperative.

Bronchodilators
- nebulized salbutomol (0.5 mg 4-hourly)
- i.v. salbutamol
- i.v. aminophylline
See Table 2.15.

Oxygen therapy
Control of inspiratory oxygen concentration is necessary to prevent hypoxia and the effects of oxygen toxicity. Therapy should commence with 24% O_2 and if the PaO_2 does not rise, use 28% O_2.

In Type II respiratory failure, oxygen therapy may cause CO_2 narcosis from the loss of hypoxic drive.

Doxapram
This is occasionally used where mechanical ventilation is contra-indicated, when $PaCO_2$ on oxygen therapy is > 10.7 kPa (80 mmHg). Doxapram infusion should take effect within 1 h and can be continued for 3-4 days at 3 mg/min.

Side effects: tachycardia; convulsions, twitching; ↑CO_2 production.

2.0 Organ failure

2.2 Respiratory failure

Mechanical ventilation
This should be considered when PaO_2 does not rise above
8 kPa(60 mmHg) with a 40% ventimask. The endotracheal tube
should have a high volume, low pressure cuff.

Optimization of ventilation/perfusion ratio can be achieved with
accurate attention to volume replacement. Monitoring RAP and
PCWP and cardiac output via a Swan-Ganz catheter will help
decide therapy with diuretics, inotropes and fluid.

PEEP should be instituted when the PaO_2 is still low on an F_1O_2
(inspired oxygen percentage) of 0.5. 2 cm H_2O PEEP should
initially be used. More than 10 cm H_2O PEEP is not recommended
as PEEP reduces venous return.

Tracheostomy is recommended if extubation cannot be considered within 10 days of commencing ventilation. Tracheostomy
should be undertaken sooner in patients who will obviously
require long-term respiratory care.

Sedation for ventilation
• opiate and relaxant e.g., phenoperidine and pancuronium given
  as intermittent i.v. boluses
• benzodiazepines
• continuous infusions of opiates, e.g. morphine (2 mg/h i.v. or
  s.c.) or omnopon (3 mg/h i.v. or s.c.). The s.c. route can be
  used with a Graseby-dynamics pump and butterfly needle sub-
  cutaneously inserted in the deltoid region.

Calculation of F_1O_2 whilst the patient is on a volume cycled
ventilator (see Fig. 2.1).

Weaning off ventilator
• it may be possible to take patients off the ventilator suddenly —
  this particularly applies to post-operative patients
• thoracic epidural may allow early weaning in chest injury
  patients
• patients who have been ventilated for a long time often benefit
  from being given gradually increasing lengths of time off the
  ventilator
• IMV (intermittent mandatory ventilation) valve — see Fig. 2.2.

Extracorporeal oxygenation
This has not come up to expectations. A recent survey has suggested that results are just as good with skilled traditional ventilation.

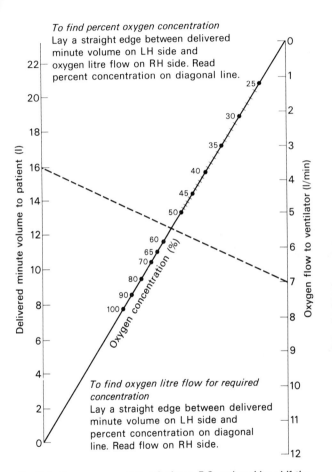

Fig. 2.1. Oxygen percentage calculator. F_IO_2 only achieved if the circuit is airtight and oxygen flow and minute volumes are acurate.

2.0 Organ failure

2.2 Respiratory failure

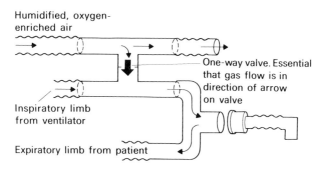

Fig. 2.2. Hudson disposable intermittent mandatory ventilation valve.

High frequency mechanical ventilation (HFMV)
There may be a place for HFMV in patients with non-compliant lungs requiring increasing PEEP and F_IO_2. As yet the circuitry has not been perfected.

Adult respiratory distress syndrome (ARDS)

Definition
Respiratory insufficiency due to interstitial pulmonary oedema resulting from increased pulmonary capillary permeability.

Severe lung oedema often precedes X-ray changes and a good end result in this syndrome depends on early treatment.

Factors predisposing to ARDS
1 Pulmonary oedema due to low COP or low serum albumin. Try to maintain serum albumin >25 g/l. N.B. Pulmonary oedema is more likely to occur if LAP (left atrial pressure as measured by PCWP in mmHg) is $>0.57 \times$ serum albumin (g/l).
2 Use of unfiltered blood—fine screen filtration should be used unless fresh blood is being transfused.
3 Organ failure
   • renal failure: may worsen fluid overload
   • liver failure: may cause lowered serum albumin
   • LVF superimposed on ARDS may be concealed without elaborate monitoring
4 Hypotension and hypovolaemia may be associated with aggregation of platelets and leucocytes which microembolize to the pulmonary microcirculation and increase vascular permeability.
5 Disseminated intravascular coagulation

2.0 Organ failure

2.2 Respiratory failure

Conditions in which ARDS is common:

Non-pulmonary
- intra-abdominal sepsis
- post shock
- head injury
- pancreatitis

Pulmonary
- pneumonia
- acid aspiration
- fat embolism

Management (see p. 41)
- early IPPV
- avoid oxygen toxicity; keep F_1O_2 <0.5
- use of PEEP 2-10 cm H_2O
- steroids in ARDS are controversial

Fat embolism syndrome

Definition
Pulmonary oedema and intra-alveolar haemorrhage due to the irritant action of unsaturated fatty acids released from fractured bones.

Clinical features
- usually a 12-72 h latent period after the fracture of pelvis or long bones
- dyspnoea
- pyrexia
- confusion
- petechial rash on chest and anterior axillary fold in 50% of patients
- Hb (haemoglobin) ↓
- platelets ↓
- DIC (disseminated intravascular coagulation) —
  definitive tests are lacking: looking for fat in sputum, urine and blood is not helpful in diagnosis
- CXR (chest X-ray) snowstorm appearance
- initial blood gas analysis ↓$PaCO_2$ ↓PaO_2

Management (see p. 41)
1 Immobilize fractured bone. Delay further surgery until pulmonary function has improved.
2 Ventilation according to criteria on p. 42.

3   Heparin therapy not universal. Consider as a continuous i.v. infusion when syndrome severe. Maintain KPTT (kaolin partial thromboplastin time 2.0-2.5 × control normal.
4   Trasylol when F_IO_2 required is >0.5.
5   Steroids controversial.
6   Antibiotics not routine. Monitor for sepsis; pyrexia and tachycardia are not reliable indicators of sepsis unless the temperature persists for 4 days.
7   Calcium serum level occasionally falls.
8   Platelets often $< 100\,000/mm^3$. Platelets rarely required.

Near drowning

In UK 1500 people die annually from drowning. Commonly their blood alcohol level is raised.

Definition
Survival after submersion. Survival following submersion for 22 min has been reported.

Clinical features
- in salt water, serum Mg^{2+} may be raised
- in fresh water, serum K^+ may be raised
- hypothermia leading to VF (ventricular fibrillation) if temp. $<30°C$
- renal failure secondary to hypoxia, acidosis, hypothermia and haemolysis

Management
All patients who have survived submersion should be admitted for observation in case they develop symptoms of secondary drowning in the first 48 h.
1   Early IPPV — see p. 41.
2   Steroids — controversial.
3   Antibiotics:
    - salt water: ampicillin + cloxacillin
    - fresh water: cephalosporin
    - swimming pool water: not indicated
4   Bronchodilators.
5   Maintain core temp. $>30°C$ (see p. 139).

6 Maintain pH > 7.2. Give 50 mmol sodium bicarbonate i.v. if pH < 7.2. Avoid sodium overload.

7 Insert RAP line. Give PPF if there is hypotension and RAP < 6 cm H_2O. If RAP > 6 cm H_2O and still hypotensive, monitor PCWP and volume; replace according to serum albumin and PCWP. Adjust ventilation to optimize CO (cardiac output).

8 Inotropes (see p. 77) indicated if hypotension and poor CO persists.

9 For severe intravascular haemolysis simple or even exchange transfusion may be necessary.

10 Secondary drowning — treat as above. If patient is already being ventilated secondary drowning rarely arises.

Pulmonary aspiration syndrome

Definition
Respiratory distress due to inhalation of acidic gastric contents. The condition should be suspected in any unconscious or anaesthetized person who vomits or regurgitates and is unable to maintain an airway. (A similar condition has been reported after aspiration of alkalis but the condition is less severe.)

Clinical features
- cyanosis
- tachypnoea
- bronchospasm
- tachycardia

Symptoms severe if pH gastric aspirate < 3.0.

Mortality is 60% and therefore *prevention* is of great importance:
- starvation prior to general anaesthesia
- regular magnesium trisilicate mixture
- presence of good suction equipment
- empty stomach with Ryle's tube
- intubation with cuffed ETT
- use of Sellick's manoeuvre when intubating somebody with a potentially full stomach

Management
1 Early IPPV (see p. 42).
2 Early endobronchial aspiration.
3 Bronchoscopy if solids aspirated. Lavage contraindicated.
4 NaHCO$_3$ i.v. if base deficit > 8 mmol.

5 Steroids—value controversial—may relieve bronchospasm.
  Advisable to give 2 doses (for litigation reasons) since still
  accepted practice.
6 Antibiotics—not used unless definite evidence of infection.
7 Antispasmodics—use with caution where oxygen reserve
  limited. May increase shunt and produce further hypoxia. If
  bronchospasm present use salbutamol or aminophylline i.v.
  (Table 2.15)

Pulmonary embolism

Clinical features
Sudden circulatory collapse with right ventricular failure and
elevated RAP. The condition is usually life-threatening when 75%
of the available pulmonary arterial tree is occluded.

Management
1 Resuscitation—ECM often propels embolism so that the initial
  total obstruction is reduced and an adequate circulatory state
  is established.
2 Inotropes—dobutamine or dopamine (p. 77-78). Noradrenaline
  often used; an excess may lead to peripheral gangrene. Run at
  rate sufficient to maintain BP>80 mmHg. If using
  noradrenaline use concentration of 4 mg/l.
3 Heparin i.v. via pulmonary artery catheter. Maintain KPTT at
  2.5 × normal; dosage very variable. Start with 10 000 iu and
  adjust between 5000 and 30 000 iu 6-hourly.
4 Thrombolytic therapy via pulmonary catheter: streptokinase
  600 000 units in 30 min then 100 000 units/h for 72 h, and
  hydrocortisone 100 mg i.v. 10 min prior to initial dose. Reso-
  lution should occur in 3 days.
  Thrombolytic therapy is contraindicated when there is:
  • operation in preceding 3 days
  • severe hypertension or preceding CVA
  • recent gastro-intestinal ulceration or haemorrhage
5 Embolectomy—requiring cardiopulmonary bypass.
  Indications:
  • BP maintenance requires increasing dose of vasopressor
  • urine production <20 ml/h
  • peripheral temperature fails to rise
  If successful, patients should be maintained on conventional
  anticoagulants for 3 months. Angiography generally preferred
  prior to surgery; should not be performed in severe shock
  unless bypass facilities available.

2.0 Organ failure

2.2 Respiratory failure

Asthma

Grading of severity
I   Can carry out job.
IA   Can carry out job with difficulty.
IB   Can carry out job with great difficulty.
II   Confined to chair; can get up.
IIA Confined to chair: can get up with difficulty.
IIB Confined to chair; can get up with great difficulty.
III   Confined to bed.
IV   Moribund.

Severe attack asthma
Clinical features
- monosyllabic speech
- thoracic over-inflation
- pulse > 120/min
- pulsus paradoxus > 10 mmHg

ECG
- RAD (right axis deviation), RVH (right ventricular hypertrophy), P pulmonale, ST changes

Spirometry
- $FEV_1 < 2$ l, PEFR < 120 l/min

Astrup
- $PaO_2 < 8$ kPa (60 mmHg)
- $PaCO_2 > 6$ kPa (45 mmHg) is a grave sign
- Metabolic acidosis

Management
1. Insert RAP, intra-arterial lines.
2. Astrup, urea and electrolytes (U&E), blood glucose (BG) level, Hb (haemoglobin), WBC (white cell count).
3. Spirometry, ECG, CXR; exclude pneumothorax.
4. Give PPF until RAP 8-10 cm H_2O.
5. Give K^+ if serum $K^+ < 4$ mmol/l.
6. O_2 by Ventimask to maintain $PaO_2 > 8.5$ kPa (64 mmHg).
7. If $PaCO_2$ in kPa $> (0.23 \times PaO_2) + 2.2$ then ventilate. (Cochrane *et al.*, 1980.)
8. Hydocortisone 4 mg/kg i.v. stat., then prednisolone 1 mg/kg i.v. 6-hourly as continuous IVI.
9. Bronchodilators. See table on p. 83.

2.0 Organ failure

2.2 Respiratory failure

10 Do aminophylline blood level if the patient has already had aminophylline.

11 Consider nebulized ipratropium 250 μg with 5 mg salbutamol 4-hourly if bronchoconstriction remains severe. If this fails, consider ether.

12 Intravenous antibiotics if specified organism identified.

Criteria for ventilation

1 Deterioration of lung function: lung collapse, pneumothorax.
- $\downarrow PaO_2 < 5.3$ kPa (40 mmHg) ⎫ exact levels decided on an
- $\uparrow PaCO_2 > 6.6$ kPa (50 mmHg) ⎭ individual patient basis
- but if $PaCO_2$ in kPa $> (0.23 \times PaO_2) + 2.2$ then IPPV should be instituted.

2 Deteriorating cardiac function
- pulse 140/min
- pulsus paradoxus
- cardiac dysrhythmias
- $\uparrow$ RAP (Suggestive but not diagnostic of RHF)

3 General deterioration
- $\downarrow$ level of consciousness
- $\downarrow$ urine output
- metabolic acidosis

4 *Bronchial lavage* using large volumes of fluid is inadvisable. Small volumes of normal saline may be used to assist removal of mucus plugs. This should be performed by skilled personnel since the manoeuvre may precipitate worsening of broncho-spasm and fatal hypoxia. Volumes of 30 ml saline (to a total of 500 ml) are squirted down each main bronchus and then removed by suction. Numerous casts can often be removed with subsequent relief of airways obstruction.

Chest injuries

Incidence
The increase in traffic on the roads has been accompanied by a sharp rise in road traffic accidents (RTA): 25% deaths from RTAs are related to chest trauma.

Chest injury may result from over-vigorous external cardiac massage following a cardiac arrest.

Definition
Flail chest results when trauma produces a double fracture of three or more adjacent ribs (see Fig. 2.3).

2.0 Organ failure

2.2 Respiratory failure

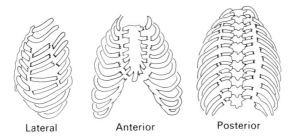

| Lateral | Anterior | Posterior |

Fig. 2.3. Types of flail chest (from Webb, 1978).

- lateral—most common
- anterior—from frontal impact; may be associated with myocardial injury and haemodynamic disturbance e.g. pericardial tamponade, hypovolaemia, sternum sucked in compressing the heart and great vessels
- posterior—the strong muscle support usually prevents any serious paradox

Lately it has been recognized that damage to the thoracic contents, including the lung parenchyma rather than the chest wall, is the factor influencing the outcome. The magnitude of the respiratory distress correlates with the extent of lung parenchymal damage and not with the extent of radiologically evident damage (see Fig. 2.4).

The concept of Pendelluft is now not thought to contribute to respiratory insufficiency.

Initial management
1 Relieve life-threatening situations:
  - clear airway
  - prevent aspiration
  - relieve pneumothorax
  - volume replacement
  - exclude pericardial tamponade
  - exclude fractures of skull, spine, pelvis
  - exclude haemorrhage, especially intracranial and intra-abdominal
  - insert RAP line in order to detect blood loss and monitor volume replacement. N.B. May read high in the presence of:
  - (a) ↑ intrathoracic pressure

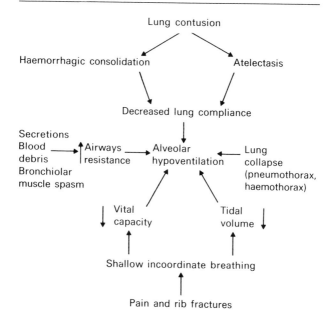

Fig. 2.4. The physiological consequences of lung trauma (from Webb, 1978).

      (b) ↑ pulmonary-vascular resistance } whilst the PCWP
      (c) pulmonary hypertension } reads low or normal
      (d) pericardial tamponade
2 Investigation:
- chest X-ray (CXR)
  - (a) include PA, lateral and oblique views, and lateral decubitus if the patient cannot sit upright
  - (b) exclude pneumothorax and haemothorax
  - (c) assess extent of flail
  - (d) watch out for development of shock-lung
- serial blood gases

Subsequent management (see Table 2.16)
1 Local anaesthetic techniques:
- intercostal blockade—requires repeated injections, useful for one or two fractured ribs
- paravertebral blockade
- thoracic epidural—patient must be conscious and able to cooperate

2.2 Respiratory failure

Epidural cannula can be left in for 1 week; perform regular top-ups.

Can use Bupivicaine or opiates. If using opiates there is always a risk of delayed respiratory arrest which responds to naloxone. These patients should therefore be kept in an ITU or on a ward capable of immediately detecting and treating a respiratory arrest.

Successful treatment of the pain of flail-chest injuries normalizes the chest movement and diminishes regional hypoventilation. It allows effective coughing and helps avoid pneumonia. After local anaesthetic, if the vital capacity is > 13 ml/kg and PaO_2 can be maintained higher than 8.5 kPa (60 mmHg), there is a strong possibility that ventilation and tracheostomy can be avoided.

2 Continuous raised airway pressure (CRAP): a modified technique for giving CRAP to patients breathing spontaneously through a tight-fitting face-mask is shown in Fig. 2.5. This may be successful if the patient is cooperative and may prevent the need for ventilation and tracheostomy.

3 Intermittent positive pressure ventilation (IPPV): only required in a minority of patients. It should only be used if there are associated severe injuries, or if there is a respiratory insufficiency (as detected clinically and by gas analysis) which does not respond to local anaesthetics, either with or without CRAP. IPPV has a significant associated morbidity and mortality. Early tracheostomy should be performed unless it is felt that the patient can be weaned off the ventilator within 7 days. The use of IMV and PEEP seems to reduce the length of time on the ventilator.

Patients may develop one of the following complications:
- ARDS
- fat embolism
- oxygen toxicity
- mediastinal subcutaneous emphysema (this rarely requires treatment)
- disseminated intravascular coagulation (DIC)
- infection
- catabolism — requires nutritional support

4 Surgery: this is indicated for the following:
- detached manubrium sterni
- ruptured trachea/bronchus
- major vessel bleed
- traumatic diaphragmatic hernia
- perforated oesophagus
- surgery for associated injuries

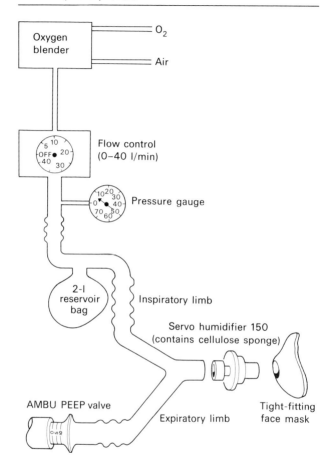

Fig. 2.5. Suggested circuit for producing continuous raised airway pressure (CRAP) in adults.

2.3   Hepatic failure

Introduction

May be:
1   Acute and superimposed on previously normal liver pathology and appears within 8 weeks of the onset of the illness, i.e. fulminant hepatic failure (FHF).
2   Develop in a patient with chronic liver disease and is commonly precipitated by various factors (see Table 2.17).

Fulminant (acute) hepatic failure
Mortality in grade IV coma (Table 2.21) is 80-90%. Causes in order of frequency are tabulated in Table 2.18. Agents which may induce fulminant hepatic failure are detailed in Table 2.19. Most patients who develop halothane hepatitis have been exposed to the agent previously. The reaction often begins with a post-operative fever associated with an eosinophilic jaundice developing 1-3 weeks post-operatively.

Hepatic failure in decompensated liver disease
The progression to coma is often slow and preceded by bizarre intellectual changes. The commonest underlying pathology is cirrhosis but liver failure may also occur in severe chronic active hepatitis, alcoholic hepatitis and extensive malignant hepatic involvement.

Clinical features

Clinical features of liver failure are listed in Table 2.20. Jaundice may be absent in very acute FHF. In cirrhosis, most patients bleed from oesophageal varices. In FHF, bleeding is generally from oesophageal or gastric erosions. A peptic ulcer may be the source of haemorrhage in both groups. Other factors contributing to the bleeding are poor hepatic synthesis of clotting factors, DIC and thrombocytopenia. Hepatic encephalopathy produces neuro-psychiatric changes; the grading is shown in Table 2.21. The mortality rate is high in patients who develop grade IV coma.

Treatment

Stop any agent/s which may have precipitated the failure (protective agents used in paracetamol intoxication should not be used when more than 8 h have elapsed after ingestion). Correct hypokalaemia and/or hypovolaemia relating to the misuse of diuretics.

Gastro-intestinal haemorrhage
Restore circulating volume with PPF or blood based on RAP serial measurements. Replace clotting factors and platelets with FFP (fresh frozen plasma) and platelet packs (see p. 97). Observe urine output and maintain careful fluid balance charts. Pass a Ryles tube. Give magnesium trisilicate mixture 2 hourly and cimetidine 200 mg i.v. 4-6 hourly in order to maintain gastric pH > 5.0.

It is important to confirm that varices are the source of bleeding by fibre optic upper gastro-intestinal (GI) endoscopy. This should be performed as soon as the patient is fit. Severe haemorrhage is often associated with portal systemic encephalopathy; an anaesthetist should therefore be present during the procedure since pulmonary aspiration is a hazard.

Medical management of variceal bleeding
1 Blood volume control is essential (see Table 3.5).
2 Give vasopressin as a continuous infusion 0.4 units/min.
3 Diarrhoea is to be expected; a serious side-effect is constriction of the coronary arteries.
4 Vasopressin is a useful temporary measure but bleeding often returns after stopping the infusion.
5 Variceal compression using a modified Sengstaken-Blakemore tube is a valuable short-term measure for controlling haemorrhage (Fig. 2.6). The upper GI tract is aspirated with a nasogastric tube and the tube removed.
6 Elevate the head of the bed approx. 10 inches and spray the pharynx with 2% lignocaine.
7 Use a new Boyce modification of the Sengstaken-Blakemore tube on each occasion and check the balloons for leaks. Ensure you know which tube connects with which oriface/balloon (Fig. 2.6).
8 With the patient in the left lateral head-up position, pass the lubricated tube into the stomach. Fill the stomach balloon with 20 ml of 20% diodone made up to 100 ml with water then with gentle traction pull the balloon up against the gastro-oesophageal junction.
9 Inflate the oesophageal balloon to 30 mmHg using a Tycos gauge. The position of the gastric balloon is then checked radiologically.
10 Once the tube is in position traction is rarely indicated. Low grade suction should be applied to the oesophageal lumen.

2.0 Organ failure

2.3 Hepatic failure

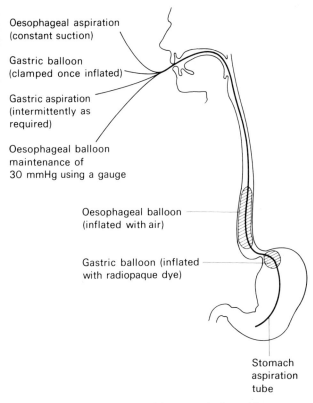

Oesophageal aspiration
(constant suction)

Gastric balloon
(clamped once inflated)

Gastric aspiration
(intermittently as
required)

Oesophageal balloon
maintenance of
30 mmHg using a gauge

Oesophageal balloon
(inflated with air)

Gastric balloon (inflated
with radiopaque dye)

Stomach
aspiration
tube

Fig. 2.6. Modified Sengstaken-Blakemore tube in position.

11 Dangers which must be observed for, and if possible
    avoided, include pulmonary aspiration, lacerations or rupture
    of the oesophagus and airway occlusion.
12 Should bleeding not be controlled by vasopressin and if
    necessary variceal compression, obliteration of the varices
    must be considered. This can be performed endoscopically or
    following trans-hepatic cannulation of the coronary vein and
    obliteration with Gelfoam or injection of a sclerosant.
13 Both the techniques require considerable expertise and the
    patient should be transferred to a unit skilled in their use.

2.0 Organ failure

2.3 Hepatic failure

Treatment of infection

1 Infection may be asymptomatic in acute onchronic hepatic failure. A source of sepsis should therefore be looked for and treated appropriately. Bronchopneumonia and primary peritonitis are remarkably common. In the presence of suspected sepsis where the source cannot be found, a four quadrant peritoneal tap is advisable. A white cell count on the ascitic fluid of greater than $1000/mm^3$ makes the diagnosis of peritonitis likely.

2 Patients with chronic liver disease have an increased susceptibility to tuberculosis.

3 Where sepsis is likely, and the organism cannot be isolated, blood cultures should be taken and the patient treated with cefuroxine and metronidazole. Where pseudonomas or proteus infection is likely, ceftazidime or gentamicin and piperacillin are the antibiotics of choice.

4 Withdrawal of alcohol in the chronic alcoholic may be complicated by withdrawal symptoms which may be confused with hepatic encephalopathy. Withdrawal symptoms are best treated by a chlormethiazole infusion, the dosage being titrated according to patient response.

Treatment of hepatic coma

1 Standard therapy is designed to reduce blood levels of nitrogenous compounds derived from the gut.

2 Protein restriction and purgation.

3 Restrict protein to 20 g of first class protein daily.

4 Magnesium sulphate enema (80 ml of a 50% solution) should be given to empty the bowel, followed by oral lactulose (see below).

5 Intestinal antibiotics. Give neomycin 1.0g orally or via a Ryles tube 6-hourly. The dosage should be revised if there is serious impairment of renal function (creatinine clearance <30% normal).

6 Lactulose syrup. Give 60 ml mane and 40 ml midday to ensure that the motions are soft and there are at least three bowel actions daily.

General measures

1 Fluid and electrolyte balance.

2 It is essential to maintain a normal circulating volume by insertion of a RAP line and maintaining the level between

4-6 cm H_2O. Volume replacement should initially be as PPF and then maintained as a dextrose solution (10-50%) with appropriate potassium replacement. Sodium ions should not be given, except to replace losses, because sodium retention is high. Amino acid preparations should be limited to 20 g of protein as pure crystalline amino acids if oral absorption is not possible. Fat emulsions should not be used.

3 Renal failure is common and has a poor prognosis when associated with acute onchronic hepatic failure but when treated appropriately may be successful in FHF. Renal failure can often be treated conservatively; when considered necessary peritoneal dialysis should be used in preference to haemodialysis.

Cardiovascular and respiratory management

1 Hypotension is common and is generally associated with a high cardiac output and low SVR. It generally responds to volume replacement but where the RAP is normal, volume replacement should be titrated against the PCWP. Where the PCWP is normal and hypotension is associated with a poor urine output (<40 ml/h), dopamine is the inotrope of choice (p. 77). Cardiac arrhythmias are common and should be treated conventionally (p. 36-37).

2 At the onset of FHF hyperventilation is common with hypocapnoea. With increasing coma, pulmonary aspiration is a risk and where there is evidence of inadequate airway control, intubation should be performed.

3 There is a high incidence of pulmonary oedema in association with liver failure—fluid and sodium overload must be avoided, the serum albumin should be maintained above 30 g with albumin infusions and the level of PCWP should be related to Se albumin or COP (p. 75).

4 There is a high incidence of bronchopneumonia, which if requiring ventilation is associated with a high mortality.

Cerebral oedema

Cerebral oedema is a common complication and is often the terminal event in liver failure—attempts at treatment have to date failed.

Temporary liver support

No system has yet been found satisfactory.

2.4   Management of renal failure

Introduction

A fall in creatinine clearance is usual in the majority of patients who are critically ill. Under certain conditions the fall is sufficiently severe to warrant special measures in order to prevent death from retention of substances normally excreted by the kidney.

Renal failure presenting in an intensive therapy unit may be acute or acute onchronic. In ARF (acute renal failure, where the kidneys are presumed to have functioned normally prior to the incident) this is generally a complication associated with severe illness. In acute onchronic renal failure some acute incident has precipitated a rapid deterioration in renal function which is already impaired.

ARF is classically divided into pre-renal, renal and post-renal. Pre-renal failure is potentially reversible and related to impaired renal perfusion. The usual response to poor perfusion is the excretion of small volumes of highly concentrated urine, which has a low sodium content (<10 mmol/l) and which contains a high urine to plasma ratio of urea and creatinine (>7.1) and a high U/P (urine/plasma) osmolality ratio (Table 2.22). Provided renal perfusion is improved, urine output will increase but should the condition be irreversible within 4 h ARF develops. Here the sodium excretion is high (>20 mmol/l) and the U/P ratio is around 1.2 (Table 2.22).

Post-renal failure
Oliguria is secondary to obstruction of the urinary tract. It must not be forgotten that partial obstruction may be associated with polyuria and it is therefore essential to exclude obstruction in all cases of renal failure.

Acute onchronic renal failure
This condition may be reversible or may proceed to an irreversible state requiring long-term dialysis. Long-standing disease should be suspected if there are any of the following features:
- pigmentation
- anaemia
- osteodystrophy
- small kidneys demonstrated by radiography or ultrasound

2.0 Organ failure

2.4 Management of renal failure

Treatment of pre-renal failure

Once pre-renal failure has been diagnosed, impaired renal perfusion must be corrected as quickly as possible.

1 Correct shock state (Section 3, p. 93).
2 Avoid Dextran 40 for volume replacement. Replace volume by
   the principle of fluid challenge should the RAP be normal.
3 Correct shock due to cardiac pathology using a drug which
   will improve renal perfusion. (Dopamine nitroprusside,
   nitroglycerine). Consider the use of digoxin.
4 Use diuretics if there is a raised LAP, *do not* use diuretics
   when hypovolaemia is suspected. Ensure Se K is normal
   before using diuretic therapy.
5 Correct hypoxia, ventilate if necessary, remembering that IPPV
   may reduce venous return and impair cardiac output. PEEP
   should be avoided if at all possible.
6 Correct metabolic imbalance. The hyperosmolar state is
   commonly associated with pre-renal failure (p. 155). In non-
   ketotic hyperosmolar coma, ARF is common. Volume replacement has to be performed extremely carefully in these patients
   since volume overload complicated by LVF is common.
   Gross changes in Se K, Ca or Mg are commonly complicated
   by a period of acute renal failure during and following correction. It is therefore essential to observe urine output and
   metabolic state carefully and to adopt the conservative
   regimen for renal failure if necessary. Treat appropriately
   hyperuricaemia (p. 154) or hypercalcaemia (p. 149).
7 Treat sepsis (being careful with dosage in potentially
   nephrotoxic antibiotics).
8 Use steroids where there has been an anaphylactic reaction.
9 Treat appropriately any overdose, in particular correct any
   metabolic, haemodynamic or oxygen deficit. Certain agents
   are known to cause renal disease and these when taken in
   excess may lead to renal failure (Table 2.23). Renal dialysis
   must be considered when renal failure is due to nephro-
   toxicity.

Treatment of post-renal failure

Post-renal failure must always be excluded in any patient with
renal failure. Features suggestive of post-renal failure have been
mentioned (p. 60). Rectal examination is essential in order to

exclude a palpable obstructive lesion. Ultrasound examination of the kidneys may be helpful.

Should the patient be sufficiently fit, a high dose IVP should be arranged immediately. Where there is fluid overload or serious metabolic imbalance (secondary to renal failure), this should be corrected prior to proceeding with an IVP.

A suspected mass in the pelvis, bladder, bowel or gynaecological pathology may necessitate diagnostic procedures once the patient is fit.

Calculus, prostatic or tumour obstruction may ultimately require removal. In order to make the patient fit enough for surgery in the presence of an obstructive lesion, the following measures may be necessary:

1 Dialysis in order to restore circulating volume and metabolic state to reasonable limits. The urea prior to surgery should be 20 mmol/l or less, the Se K 4.5 mmol/l or less and the patient normovolaemic. Generally the Hb is restored to 8.0-10.0 g prior to surgery.
2 Pre-operatively give two to three packs of FFP and insert a RAP line (if not already present). Check the platelet count and if $<80\,000/mm^3$ give four packs of platelets pre-operatively and during the operation.
3 Give appropriate antibiotic therapy if sepsis is present.
4 During operation the patient should be hyperventilated, hypoxia and fluid overload avoided. Blood should be as fresh as possible and a dangerous rise in Se K avoided by using the dextrose/insulin regime (100 ml 50% dextrose + actrapid insulin according to blood glucose).
5 Be prepared to ventilate the patient postoperatively.
6 Be prepared to dialyse postoperatively, if renal function does not return rapidly.
7 Commonly the patient becomes polyuric post relief of an obstruction — maintenance of fluid and electrolyte balance is essential. Metabolic balance is made easier by analysing the urine and any other aspirate for electrolytes. Observe for sodium and potassium depletion.
8 Under certain circumstances (e.g. following calculus removal in a unilateral kidney), where renal function is not restored adequately, long-term dialysis has to be considered.

2.0 Organ failure

2.4 Management of renal failure

Management of ARF

There are many factors which may precipitate ARF, the most important of which are listed in Table 2.24.

It is essential in the critically ill to make the diagnosis early since these patients are catabolic and death from hyperkalaemia can occur within 48 h of the onset of ARF.

Once the diagnosis has been made, establish the conservative regime for ARF.

Fluids, electrolytes and nutrition
Once normovolaemia has been achieved (by titration of fluid volume against the RAP), fluids should be restricted to 300 ml plus the previous day's urine output. Allowances must be made for GI secretions (p. 178), sweating (p. 243), and hyperventilation.

Sodium ions should not be replaced unless there are heavy losses and serum potassium can often be maintained within the normal range using the dextrose insulin regimen.

Usual fluid is 20-50% dextrose intravenously giving 200-500 g carbohydrate daily. Glucose intolerance is common and BG > 10.0 mmol will require the addition of actrapid insulin.

Carbohydrate can be given orally as hycal or as caloreen down the Ryles tube. Fat is generally not used as an initial calorific source since intolerance is common.

Potassium is not given. Blood, if absolutely necessary, should be as fresh as possible.

First class protein is given as 0.5 g protein/kg BW daily as Vamin glucose, Albumaid down the Ryles tube or as two eggs daily.

Treatment of complications
1 Fluid overload should not be allowed to occur but when present generally requires dialysis.
2 Hyperkalaemia (see Table 4.15). The quickest regime is dextrose and insulin giving initially 100 ml 50% dextrose + 12 units actrapid insulin intravenously over 15 min.
3 Calcium chloride should be given if there is a serious cardiac dysrhythmia. These measures are temporary and are generally followed by dialysis.

2.0 Organ failure

2.4 Management of renal failure

4 Haemorrhage — patients with ARF are predisposed to GI haemorrhage, commonly secondary to stress. Early regular antacid therapy (with aluminium hydroxide) may cut down the incidence. We prefer not to use H_2 antagonists since there seems to be an increased risk of thrombocytopenia with their use.

5 Anaemia — patients tend to get progressively anaemic. The haemoglobin level is generally maintained between 7-8 g/dl unless the condition is acute onchronic renal failure, when it may be allowed to fall lower.

6 Infection — patients with ARF are predisposed to super-infection; prophylactic antibiotics must not be used. A fever developing in a patient with ARF is an indication to culture all suspected sources of infection and to remove any catheters which may be the source of sepsis (e.g. RAP line, urinary catheter, peritoneal dialysis catheter). Antibiotic dosage must be carefully regulated.

7 Organ failure — failure of other organs is common in any patient who has had a period of shock and should be treated appropriately. Hypoxia is common, patients with ARF being particularly predisposed to the shock lung syndrome. IPPV is commonly required.

Specific treatment
1 Renal failure secondary to toxicity of certain agents may be an indication for early dialysis.

2 Obstruction should be relieved as soon as the patient is fit enough for the relevant operative procedure.

3 Where ARF is thought to be due to intrinsic autoimmune disease, a renal biopsy should be performed as soon as the patient is fit. Under such circumstances a nephrological opinion must be obtained since it may be considered appropriate to use steroids and immunosuppressives before the renal biopsy has been performed.

4 Symmetrically enlarged kidneys with no evidence of obstruction may be secondary to infiltrative disease (reticulosis, leukaemia, amyloidosis) and an early biopsy may be indicated if the disease cannot be detected by other means.

Renal dialysis
1 Indication — the decision to dialyse the patient has to be undertaken on an individual basis and should be made by a clinician experienced in its use.

2 Early dialysis (BU < 25 mmol) — this will be performed generally under the following circumstances:

2.4 Management of renal failure

- hypercatabolism (BU rise greater than 10 mmol/24 h)
- high serum potassium for other reasons, e.g. haemolysis
- renal failure thought to be due to a dialysable agent (e.g. amino glycosides)
- where biochemical and haematological indices have to be brought down to near normal levels for surgery or renal biopsy
- presence of complications, e.g. fluid overload.
- where fluid has to be given, e.g. blood with the possible complication of fluid overload

3 Late dialysis (BU allowed to rise 25-40 mmol/l — conditions where the period of acute renal failure is likely to be short:
  - e.g. gross metabolic changes — cardiac conditions where the hazard of dialysis may be associated with an increased mortality:
  - renal failure secondary to cardiac disease
  - renal failure secondary to hepatic disease
  - the hypocatabolic patient (BU rise generally <5 mmol/24 h)

4 Type of dialysis — this may be governed by several factors:
  - availability of haemodialysis
  - preference of the clinician
  - patient's age
  - underlying cause for ARF
  - suitability of the peritoneum
  - contrasting efficiency of the two systems

The decision should be made by a clinician skilled in the management of ARF. Peritoneal dialysis is the preferable system for the young, the elderly and the patient with haemodynamic instability. It may not be sufficiently efficient in the severely catabolic patient and cannot be used when there is a leaky peritoneal cavity (e.g. multiple fistulae, pelvic surgery), or the peritoneal cavity is unsuitable (e.g. multiple bowel adhesions). Peritoneal dialysis can be used in the presence of intraperitoneal sepsis. Haemodialysis may be the preferable system in rare circumstances when efficient dialysis of toxins is essential.

5 Dialysis technique will not be discussed.

6 During dialysis certain factors have to be closely observed:
  - fluid balance (RAP monitoring, daily weighing)
  - metabolic balance — Se K must be observed carefully. A fall in Se Na generally implies water overload unless there are overt Na losses
  - nutritional state — high calorie intake essential. During dialysis protein administration may be increased (40-80 g daily)

2.0 Organ failure

2.4 Management of renal failure

- ventilatory care — patients on peritoneal dialysis are particularly predisposed to basal atelectasis
- haematological state — blood is generally required especially in the catabolic patient. Thrombocytopenia — clotting factor deficits rarely require treatment except if the patient is due for operation
- drugs — drugs excreted by the kidney should be avoided or used in reduced dosage. Sedation is preferably given by a reversible drug, e.g. opiates. Nephrotoxic antibiotic dosage must be regulated according to blood levels — tetracycline must *not* be used

7 Antacids — these are generally given as aluminium hydroxide (magnesium trisilicate raises the Se Mg). Aluminium blood levels should be observed. H_2 antagonists are generally not required.

8 Vitamins — folic acid and B_{12} must be replaced in adequate dosage.

9 *Operation* — many patients on dialysis will require surgery. Ensure that any deficit in clotting is corrected, circulating volume is low normal, Se K around 3.5 mmol/l, appropriate anaesthesia is given and that facilities are available to ventilate postoperatively. In a catabolic patient in ARF the major cause may be sepsis requiring urgent surgery. Here, the operation should be covered with a dextrose insulin regimen and the patient hyperventilated during the procedure. Should the source of sepsis be intraperitoneal, a dialysing catheter can be put in under direct vision during the operation. It is preferable to defer dialysis until 24 h postoperatively in order to ensure haemodynamic stability.

10 Dialysis and the hypercatabolic patient — death in these patients is commonly due to hyperkalaemia. In the presence of a haemodynamically unstable patient, peritoneal dialysis can be introduced for the first 2-3 days, changing to haemodialysis if the Se creatinine is not contained.

Recovery following ARF

With careful control of fluid balance there is rarely a diuretic response, urine output slowly increasing. Once urine output is > 1.0 l/day the conservative regimen can generally be adopted. Daily estimation of urinary area, creatinine, Na and K, is essential since the patient may be polyuric and yet creatinine clearance be inadequate.

During the recovery phase observe for dehydration, sodium and potassium depletion.

2.0   Organ failure

2.5   Tables

Table 2.1. Treatment of cardiac arrest

Phase I
1 If patient connected to drips or suction, place board on bed and roll patient on to it. The floor is preferable
2 Lower the head and clear the airway
3 Raise the legs
4 Thump middle of sternum once

Phase II
1 Begin closed chest massage
2 Mouth-to-mouth respiration—an Ambu bag, rebreathing bag connected to air or oxygen, or a Brooke airway should be used if possible
3 Send for assistance *once instituted*

Phase III
1 Intubate the trachea
2 Erect an intravenous drip
3 Record an ECG

Phase IV—Definitive treatment
1 50 mmol sodium bicarbonate i.v.
2 5 ml 10% calcium chloride (0.45 mmol Ca^{2+}/ml) via drip tubing
3 1 ml 1:1000 adrenaline hydrochloride via drip tubing if small magnitude VF is present
4 Defibrillate externally or apply the pacemaker as necessary. If an ECG trace cannot be obtained quickly, defibrillate blind
5 Following cardioversion, commence lignocaine infusion 1-2 mg/min following a loading dose 60-120 mg
6 Asystole. Attempt to obtain VF with intracardiac adrenaline. Treat precipitating factor(s) if possible

Phase V—Supportive treatment
1 Consider ventilation initially with FiO_2 1.0, then subsequently maintain PaO_2 9.3—13.3 kPa (70-100 mmHg) and $PaCO_2$ 3.7—4.0 kPa (28-30 mmHG)
2 Check Se K and if >4.5 mmol/l give dexamethasone 4 mg i.v.
3 Check RAP and if <5 cm H_2O give mannitol 20% 2 g/kg over 10 min
4 Catheterize the bladder—observe urine output
5 Check acid base and electrolyte balance and correct if necessary
6 Keep the patient cool 33-35°C

Table 2.2. Immediate post-arrest management

I   Cardiac
1   Sustained low BP and poor urine output: consider an
     inotrope (Table 2.9 p. 78)
2   Pulse rate <60/min: consider cardiac pacing
3   Multiform ventricular extrasystoles: use an antidysrhythmic
     (Table 2.8 p. 76)
4   Exclude a metabolic abnormality—hypoxia, hypovolaemia,
     cardiac failure or cardiac tamponade
5   Where there is a potentially correctable surgical lesion,
     consider transfer to a cardiac unit for urgent investigation.
     Balloon counterpulsation may be of value in maintaining
     cardiac output (CO) in the presence of cardiogenic shock

II   Respiratory
1   *Do not* extubate should factors be present which may
     produce respiratory difficulty
2   Should IPPV or CPPV be indicated:
        Maintain PaO_2 9.3-13.3 kPa (70-100 mmHg) $PaCO_2$ at
        3.7-4.0 kPa (28-30 mmHg)
        Treat pulmonary aspiration
        Treat extensive chest trauma

III   Cerebral
1   If period of arrest prior to resuscitation is >2 min or
     resuscitation lasts >15 min give mannitol 100 ml 15% i.v.
     and dexamethasone 4 mg i.v., continue dexamethasone
     4 mg i.m. 6-hourly for three doses.
2   Hyperventilate and maintain $PaCO_2$ 3.7-4.0 kPa
     (28-30 mmHg)

Table 2.3. Factors which may contribute to or precipitate a cardiac dysrhythmia

These include:

Metabolic abnormalities	— changes in K^+ Ca^{2+} Mg^{2+} acid base
Respiratory abnormalities	— changes in PaO_2 $PaCO_2$
Pulmonary abnormalities	— factors producing mediastinal shift, pulmonary non-compliance, increasing airway pressures
Cardiac abnormalities	— cardiac ischaemia, failure, valvular abnormalities, myocardial disease (e.g. myocarditis), cardiac tamponade
Hypertensive heart disease	
Sepsis — in particular	— septicaemia and shock peritonitis cholecystitis bacterial endocarditis
Pancreatitis	
Endocrine disease	— thyroid disease phaeochromocytoma
Renal failure	
Hepatocellular failure	
Diseases of the CNS (central nervous system)	— raised ICP meningitis brain stem abnormalities Guillain-Barré syndrome tetanus
Stress	
Pain	
Drugs — in particular	— digoxin, tricyclic antidepressants

Table 2.4. Parenteral anti-arrhythmic drugs most commonly used in the ITU

Drug	Dosage	Indications	Comments
β-blockers			
Propranolol	1-10 mg slow i.v. (1 mg/min)	Phaeochromocytoma Thyrotoxicosis	Cardioselective Non-cardioselective Potent myocardial depressant
Practolol	5-20 mg slow i.v.	Arrhythmias due to mitral valve prolapse Anaesthetic arrhythmias May be considered very rarely in intoxication due to digoxin (in the absence of A-V block) and tricyclic antidepressants	Cardioselective Should not be used orally Generally avoided in the critically ill because of the potent negative inotropic effect. Do not use either drug in the patient with history of bronchospasm.
Calcium antagonist			
Verapamil	i.v. infusion 1 mg/min to a total of 10 mg i.v. bolus 5-10 mg repeated after 10 min then 0.005 mg/kg/min if needed as	SVT	Negligible effect on ventricular arrhythmias Do not use when there is impaired sinus node function or A-V conduction defects

	In myocardial disease, β-blockade, digitalis intoxication, start at 0.001 mg/kg/min, increase gradually titrating against heart rate		
Membrane stabilizing agents			
Lignocaine	50-100 mg slow i.v. repeated once or twice at 5-10 min intervals followed by infusion if necessary 1-4 mg/min	Drug of choice for ventricular ectopics or runs of VT (ventricular tachycardia)	Use with care in A-V block. Overdose may produce agitation and convulsions
Tocainide	500-750 mg i.v. infused over 15-30 min followed immediately by 600-800 mg orally	Similar activity to lignocaine of equal value, provided patient able to take tablets orally	Same as lignocaine
Disopyramide	2 mg/kg (not >150 mg) i.v. slowly over 5 min then oral therapy or a slow infusion of 20-30 mg/h (0.4 mg/kg/h) to a maximum 800 mg/24 h	Control of ventricular dysrhythmias. Less frequently used for supraventricular dysrhythmias. Dysrhythmias associated with the WPW Syndrome	Reduce dosage in the presence of renal failure. Disopyramide blood levels preferable in the presence of renal failure
Mexilitine	150 mg i.v. over 5 min followed by an infusion given at a rate of	Control of ventricular arrhythmias	Nausea, vomiting, drowsiness may occur with overdosage;

continued

Table 2.4—*continued*

	250 mg/30 min, then 250 mg over 150 min, then 500 mg over 8 h. Subsequently 500 mg/12 h. Additional doses of 50-100 mg i.v. may be given; the infusion rate must *not be* changed		symptoms subside with dosage reduction
Procainamide	i.v. 50 mg/min to a total of 1.0 g May be given i.m.	Ventricular dysrhythmias	Observe for hypotension Avoid in renal or hepatic failure *Should not be* used long term May cause hypotension
Phenytoin	100 mg bolus via a 5% dextrose infusion over 2 min to a total of 1.0 g	Ventricular dysrhythmias	Avoid in patients with A-V block

Agents widening action—potential duration (major effect)

Amiodarone	5 mg/kg BW in 100 ml 5% dextrose i.v. over 15 min then adjust according to response up to 1000 mg/24 h	Tachyarrhythmias may be used in bundle branch block with A-V conduction disorders	Initial hypotension usual *Do not* give too rapidly Avoid in the presence of β-blockers; calcium antagonists may potentiate a brachycardia Use with caution in the presence of digoxin
Digitalis	Digoxin i.v. loading dose 0.75 mg, in the acutely ill reduce to 0.5 mg This is repeated 2-4 h later	Congestive cardiac failure and AF Uncontrolled AF	Avoid in heart block, hypertrophic obstructive cardiomyopathy, certain cases of WPW syndrome and hypokalaemia Monitor blood levels in the critically ill For factors affecting digitalis sensitivity see Table 2.7 p. 75

Table 2.5. Atrial rate, A-V conduction and response to carotid sinus massage

Rhythm	Atrial rate	A-V conduction	Effect of carotid sinus massage
Sinus tachycardia	100-200 Rarely > 150	1:1	Slows
Atrial tachycardia	140-240	Usually 2:1 Slower rates may be 1:1	Nil May increase A-V block
Proxysmal nodal tachycardia	140-240	Variable block arises in A-V junction	Nil or may stop
Non-proxysmal junctional tachycardia	60-140	Variable Arises in A-V junction	Ventricular rate may slow
WPW syndrome	140-240	1:1	Nil or may stop
Atrial flutter	250-350	Variable block generally 2:1, rarely 1:1	Nil or increases block making diagnosis easier Occasionally changes to AF
Atrial fibrillation (AF)	> 350	Variable	Ventricular rate may slow

Table 2.6. Treatment of SVT

		Treatment
1	Sinus tachycardia	Nil. Treat underlying cause
2	Paroxysmal SVT	
	Atrial tachycardia	Consider carotid sinus massage
	Paroxysmal nodal tachycardia	Consider digoxin
		Consider intravenous β-blockade
	Atrial flutter	if patient already on digoxin

		Consider verapamil if patient *not* on digoxin, should patient be in cardiogenic shock for d.c. cardioversion or rapid atrial pacing
3	Atrial fibrillation	Digoxin usual treatment, alternatives are practolol or verapamil
		d.c. cardioversion should the patient be in cardiogenic shock
		Consider anticoagulant therapy
4	Non-paroxysmal junctional tachycardia	Usually no treatment required
		Consider: atropine
		atrial pacing
		isoprenaline

Table 2.7. Factors altering digoxin therapeutic efficacy

Generalized disorders
Renal failure (diminishing excretion)
Chronic cardiac disease (impaired intracellular Ca ion transport)
Chronic pulmonary disease (hypoxia acid base changes)
Acute hypoxia (sensitive to digitalis-induced dysrhythmias)
Hyperthyroidism (increases half life)
Low muscle mass (reduced digitalis muscle binding)

Cardiac disorders
Acute myocardial infarction—? increased sensitivity
Acute rheumatic heart disease—increased sensitivity
Chronic IHD ⎫
Thyrotoxicosis ⎭ —decreased sensitivity

Electrolyte imbalance
Hyperkalaemia, hyponatraemia, hypovolaemia—decreased sensitivity
Hypokalaemia, hypomagnesaemia, hypercalcaemia—increased sensitivity

Drug therapy
Quinidine—reduce digitalis dosage by half
β-blockers (verapamil)—majority increase A-V block
Barbiturates, phenylbutazone, phenytoin—decrease blood levels

Table 2.8. Treatment of ventricular tachyarrhythmias

		Treatment	
1	Accelerated idioventricular rhythm	No treatment unless haemodynamic performance impaired	
		Rates 60-90/min:	atropine i.v. atrial pacing
		Rates 90-120/min:	lignocaine disopyramide mexilitine
2	Ventricular tachycardia Torsade de pointes (variant of ventricular tachycardia)	Exclude aetiological factors	
		Deteriorating haemodynamic state:	d.c. shock
		Otherwise choose from:	lignocaine mexilitine disopyramide phenytoin bretylium procainamide tocainide amiodarone
		Drugs less commonly used:	

2.0 Organ failure

2.5 Tables

Table 2.9. Some drugs used in cardiac failure

	Drug	Dosage	Indications	Comments
Diuretics	Frusemide	40-250 mg i.v. >120 mg as an infusion	Pulmonary oedema Biventricular failure	Ensure normal Se K Avoid swinging from hyper-volaemia to hypovolaemia Frusemide venodilator
	Bumetamide	1-5 mg i.v. >2 mg as an infusion		
Opiates	Diamorphine Papavaretum	2.5-10 mg iv. 5-20 mg i.v.	Acute anxiety and pulmonary oedema	Titrate i.v. very slowly, avoid respiratory depression, observe for hypotension *Do not use* if BP SP 110 or less or pulse rate <80/min Venodilators
Inotropes Cardiac glycosides	Digoxin	0.25-0.5 mg i.v. slow titration	Pulmonary oedema with atrial flutter or fibrillation Consider in LVF in patients with SVT	Avoid where KI, suspected digoxin toxicity, presence of A-V block In acute situation, especially in the presence of renal failure, monitor digoxin blood level
	Dopamine hydrochloride	0.5-30 μg/kg/min as an infusion	Cardiogenic shock with hypotension and anuria	May increase heart rate High doses α-adrenergic effect—

continued

77

2.5 Tables

Table 2.9—*continued*

	Dobutamine	0.5-10 μg/kg/min as an infusion	Cardiogenic shock in the presence of ↑SVR	not >4 μg/kg if there is increase in SVR or use dobutamine instead Stop increase in the presence of increasing SVR and consider combining with dobutamine Does not increase renal perfusion May increase heart rate
	Isoprenaline hydrochloride	0.5-10 μg/min as an infusion	Cardiogenic shock with bradycardia and SVR↑	Dangerous increase in heart rate May be valuable in very low dosage with dopamine or dobutamine
Peripheral vasodilators	Hydralazine	Test dose 2.5-5.0 mg i.v. as test dose—if BP SP does not fall BP SP >90 mmHg give infusion of 7.5 mg every 4-6 h (improvement within 8 h)	Pulmonary oedema especially in the presence of hypertension and SVR↑	Avoid with BP SP <90 mm Increases pulse rate Arteriolar dilator Does *not* alter LVFP (left ventricular filling pressure)

Isosorbide dinitrate	1-10 mg hourly as an infusion	Pulmonary oedema especially in the presence of recent myocardial ischaemia	Avoid with BP SP <90 mm Increase pulse rate, increases renal perfusion, improves coronary perfusion, myocardial oxygen sparing Venular dilator may be combined with hydrallazine Reduces LVFP but does not reduce SVR
Nitroprusside	0.5-1.5 μg/kg/min as an infusion	Pulmonary oedema with high SVR especially when its use is likely to be required for <24 h	Avoid use BP SP <90 mmHg Inc. pulse rate Improves coronary perfusion < isosorbide dinitrate Arteriolar and venular dilator Reduces SVR Do not infuse for longer than 24 h Reduces LVFP

Table 2.10. Drugs used in the treatment of severe hypertension which requires urgent and controlled depression

	Dosage	Side effects	Comments
After-load reducer Hydralazine	100 mg/100 ml 1/5 n saline Infuse at a rate of 10 mg every 15 min and stop once required BP achieved Continuous infusion 20-100 mg 12-hourly to control BP	Tachyphylaxis Tachycardia Avoid if circulating blood volume low	Top up essential if circulating blood volume low Avoid in patients with pulse rate >110/min
Nitroprusside	Infusion solution with 5% dextrose rate 0.5-1.5 μg/kg/min until satisfactory BP achieved, then adjust maintenance 0.5-0.8 μg/kg/min—max. infusion rate 800 μg/min	Preferable not to use >72 h Avoid use in the elderly Contraindicated in pregnancy	Volume controlled infusion and continuous intra-arterial monitoring essential
α- and β-blocker Labetolol	200 mg in 100 ml 1/5 n saline Infuse at rate of 2 mg/min continuous monitoring of BP and stop infusion once desirable effect achieved (dosage generally 50-300 mg) Maintenance dosage generally 50-100 mg 8-12 hourly	Rarely produces bradycardia May exacerbate cardiac failure and ↓CO	Useful in patients with tachycardia Ensure adequate circulating blood volume

2.0 Organ failure

Table 2.11. Procedure for lowering acute severe hypertension

Monitor
  Intra-arterial BP
  RAP
  Skin/core temperature differential
  Where LAP is in doubt insert a PCWP as soon as possible
  Hourly urine output

Drugs
  Select most appropriate drug (see Table 2.10 p. 80)

Postoperative patient
  Intravenous nitroprusside for 24-48 h followed by oral therapy
  generally appropriate

Patient with LV overload
  Consider nitroprusside or hydrallazine + diuretics

Patient with tachycardia and severe stress with good myocardial
function and normal PCWP
  Consider labetolol
  e.g. phaeochromocytoma, recent cerebral catastrophe,
  eclampsia, pre-eclampsia, certain postoperative cases

On occasions the combination of hydrallazine and labetolol has
proven useful

Table 2.12. Causes of respiratory failure

Respiratory centre involvement
  Infiltration or Compression
  Depression, Haemorrhage
  Neoplasia, Trauma
  Metabolic Drugs

High cervical cord involvement
  Infiltration
  Compression

Neuromuscular juction derangement
  Myasthenia gravis
  Muscle relaxants
  Aminoglycosides   *continued*

Table 2.12—*continued*

Motor nerve involvement
  Poliomyelitis
  Peripheral neuritis
  Motor neurone disease
  High spinal/epidural

Muscular disorders
  Dystrophia myotonica

Chest wall involvement
  Trauma

Parenchymal lung disease
  Pneumothorax
  Pneumonia

Airway involvement
  Obstruction e.g. tumour
  Constriction e.g. asthma

Contributory factors
  Postoperative pain
  Obesity
  Peritonitis
  Pancreatitis
  LVF

Table 2.13. Immediate postoperative respiratory failure

Obstruction or mechanical problem

CNS depression
  Drugs
  Hypocapnia following hyperventilation

Suxamethonium apnoea

Residual curarization
  too little neostigmine
  myasthenia gravis
  aminoglycosides
  acidosis

Malignant hyperpyrexia

CO_2 narcosis

Table 2.14. Physiotherapy: position of the patient for drainage of various lung segments

Affected lobe		Position
Lingula		Supine, head-down
Middle lobe		
L. lateral basal		R. lateral
Lower lobe	apical segment	Prone, head-down
	anterior basal	R. lateral, head-down
R. upper lobe		Tilt to L., head-up
L. upper lobe		Tilt to R., head-down

Table 2.15. Recommended dosage of aminophylline and salbutamol given intravenously

	Dosage of i.v. aminophylline		
	Loading-dose (mg/kg over 20 min)	Maintenance (mg/kg/h)	Plasma level (mg/1)
Children			
low dose	6	1.10	10
high dose	9	1.65	15
Adults			
low dose	6	0.90	10
high dose	9	1.35	15

Toxicity: when plasma level >20 mg/1, there is anorexia, abdominal pain, nausea, vomiting, ventricular ectopics.
Prevention: reduce dose by one third in heart failure, by one half in liver failure, by one half if already on *oral theophylline*
Treatment: discontinue aminophylline; consider practolol i.v. valium

Dosage of i.v. salbutamol	
Loading-dose (μg/kg over 20 min)	Maintenance (μg/kg/min)
4	0.05-0.3

Table 2.16. Classification of injuries*

Grade	Clinical features	Treatment
1—mild	Few fractured ribs; adequate cough; no ventilatory impairment; $PaCO_2\downarrow$; PaO_2 normal or slightly$\downarrow$	Humidified oxygen percentage appropriate to lung condition and pain relief by local anaesthetic, regional blockade, or analgesic drugs
2—moderate	Possible flail segment; inadequate cough; ventilatory impairment; $PaCO_2\downarrow$; PaO_2 generally$\downarrow$; other injuries fairly common	Consider regional blockade; consider tracheostomy (mandatory in chronic lung disease) humidified oxygen percentage appropriate to lung condition; IPPV probably necessary
3—severe	Flail segment as in grade 2; $PaCO_2\downarrow$; $PaO_2\downarrow$; other injuries common	Tracheostomy; IPPV; oxygen percentage administered appropriate to lung condition

*Reproduced with kind permission of Webb (1978)

Table 2.17. Factors precipitating hepatic failure in chronic liver disease

Inappropriate use of sedatives and analgesics
Misuse of diuretics
Gastro-intestinal haemorrhage
Infection
Alcohol consumption

Table 2.18. Causes of FHF (in order of frequency)

Acute viral hepatitis
Paracetamol overdose
Halothane associated
Other drugs (see Table 2.19)
Acute fatty liver of pregnancy
Mushroom poisoning (amanita phalloides)
Leptospirosis

Table 2.19. Agents which may cause hepatocellular necrosis

Antidepressant	Monoamine-oxidase inhibitors
Antimicrobials	Isoniazid
	Pyrazinamide
	Ethionamide
	PAS
	Sulphonamides
	Nitrofurantoin
	Tetracycline
Anticonvulsants	Phenytoin
Antispasmodics	Dantrolene
Anaesthetics	Halothane
	Methoxyflurane
	Fluroxene

Table 2.20. Clinical features of liver failure

Jaundice	Hepatic encephalopathy
Haemorrhagic tendency	Abnormalities in glucose metabolism
Ascites*	Other endocrine disturbances*
Fluid retention	Altered drug metabolism
Renal failure	Osteomalacia and osteoporosis*

*Manifestations of hepatic failure in decompensated liver disease.

Table 2.21. Grading of hepatic encephalopathy

Grade 1
  Euphoria, occasional depression
  Fluctuant mild confusion
  Slowness of mentation and effect
  Untidy, slurred speech
  Disordered sleep rhythm

Grade II
  Drowsy but responds to simple commands
  Inappropriate behaviour

Grade III
  Sleeps most of the time—rousable
  Marked confusion
  Speech incoherent

Grade IV
  Unrousable
  Muscle flaccidity
  Decerebrate or grand mal convulsions

Table 2.22. Differential diagnosis of oliguria based on U/P osmolality ratio

Aetiology	U/P osmolality ratio
Dehydration	2.7-4.0
Poor perfusion	2.0-1.3
Acute intrinsic renal failure	<1.2

Table 2.23. Drugs which may cause renal failure

Pre-renal failure

Diuretics	↑	dehydration
Laxatives		
Tetracyclines	↑	inc. urine Na excretion
		catabolism
		polyuria

Post-renal failure (obstructive uropathy)

Anticoagulants	↑	retroperitoneal haemorrhage
Cytotoxics	↑	uric acid
6MP		
Methotrexate	↑	crystalluria
Acetazolamide		
Sulphonamides		
Myeloma	↑	Bence Jones protein
Intravascular haemolysis	↑	haemoglobin
Vit. D preparations		
Acetazolamide	↑	calcium deposition
Hypervitaminosis A		
Milk alkali syndrome		
Silicates	↑	silicon deposition
Papillary necrosis	↑	analgesic abuse, aspirin/phanacetin aspirin/paracetamol combinations, phenacetin

continued

Table 2.23—*continued*

Glomerular damage

Nephrotic syndrome → gold
penicillamine

Drug-induced LE syndrome → large number of drugs, in particular hydralazine, INAH, procainamide; severe renal failure unusual

Interstitial and tubular damage

Interstitial nephritis → penicillin therapy
sulphonamides
phenindione
rifampicin
thiazides
frusemide

Acute tubular necrosis commonest cause for drug-induced renal failure

Aminoglycosides
Polymyxins
Cephalosporins—cephaloridine
Amphotericin B
⎫
⎬ ↑ may be precipitated by the use of frusemide
⎭

Analgesics—paracetamol, aspirin

Radiological contrast media—particularly likely to occur in the presence of hepatocellular dysfunction and dehydration

2.5 Tables

Table 2.24. The most common conditions giving rise to ARF

Multiple trauma
Septicaemia

Sepsis in particular $\begin{cases} \text{pneumonia} \\ \text{cholecystitis} \end{cases}$

Gastric or bowel surgery
Ruptured or dissecting aortic aneurysm
Acute pancreatitis
Metabolic—in particular K↓ Ca↑ uric acid↑
Post-myocardial infarction
Drug overdose and drug toxicity
Pulmonary embolism
Post-cardiopulmonary bypass
Burns
Obstetric
Autoimmune

2.6 References

Cochrane G. M., Prior J. G. & Wolff C. B. (1980) Chronic stable asthma and the normal arterial pressure of carbondioxide in hypoxia. *Brit. Med. J.* **281**, 705.

Mellemgraad K. (1966) Alveolar-arterial oxygen difference: its size and components in normal man. *Acta. Physiol. Scand.* **67**, 10.

Pitcher J. (1982) Inserting a temporary pacemaker. *Medicine* **1**, 814.

Webb A. K. (1978) Flail chest - management and complications. *Brit. J. Hosp. Med.* **20**, 406.

Yacoub M. H. (1978) Mechanical circulatory support using intra-aortic balloon counterpulsation. In *Medical Management of the Critically Ill Patient* (Ed. by G. C. Hanson & P. L. Wright), p. 955. Academic Press, London.

2.0 Organ failure

Notes

2.0 Organ failure

Notes

3.0   Shock

3.1   Definition, 95

3.2   Pathophysiology, 95

3.3   Shock due to changes in circulating blood volume, 95
Shock and fluid overload
Shock and hypovolaemia
Treatment of shock due to decrease in circulating volume
Management of haemorrhagic shock

3.4   Particular aspects of trauma, 98
Introduction
Management of head injuries
Management of spinal injuries
Management of a cervical injury
Management of abdominal injuries
Management of burns
Management of injuries of the genito-urinary tract
Management of electrical and lightning injuries

3.5   Shock and sepsis, 102
Introduction
General management
Sequential management
Unusual types of shock and sepsis

3.6   Tables, 114

3.7   References, 134

3.0 Shock

3.1 Definition / 3.2 Pathophysiology / 3.3 Circulation

3.1 Definition

Shock is a condition characterized by a disordered haemodynamic state with associated evidence of inadequate organ perfusion.

3.2 Pathophysiology

Various mechanisms can result in shock, the most obvious being pump failure, obstruction in the main channel of flow, e.g. massive pulmonary embolism and depletion of circulating blood volume. Shock associated with sepsis is complex and the pathophysiological mechanisms producing shock variable. Certain areas of the body are affected to a greater or lesser degree in all forms of shock — the microcirculation, rheological and coagulative properties of blood, the heart and vital organs (Hanson, 1978[1]).

3.3 Shock due to changes in circulating blood volume

Shock and fluid overload

It must not be forgotten that overload of the circulation may lead to cardiac and pulmonary failure and shock. Treatment must be directed to management of the cause (Table 3.1).

Shock and hypovolaemia

Shock secondary to a decrease in circulating blood volume may be due to various causes (Table 3.2) and on occasions is very complex, e.g. epidural blockade and obstetric haemorrhage. The majority of these causes have been discussed in other chapters (renal failure, p. 60, salt and water loss, p. 144).

Treatment of shock due to decrease in circulating volume

Choice of fluids for volume replacement
In acute conditions the rate and volume of replacement is more important than the type of fluid given. Clearly, in metabolic problems the fluid selected would depend upon the predominant deficit.

In patients where more than one third of the blood volume is lost acutely, or where there is repeated blood volume loss, or the

3.3 Changes in circulating blood volume

serum albumin is likely to be low already, the fluid should be carefully selected because (1) the serum albumin will fall unless albumin-containing solutions are used, (2) as a result maintenance of intra-vascular volume will require a greater volume of crystalloid in relation to the volume lost and there will be an increased tendency towards interstitial oedema.

Literature has shown (Hauser *et al.*, 1980), that under such circumstances fluid volume replacement should be with an oncotic solution (dextran 70 haemaccel) with a protein-containing solution (PPF or 25% salt poor albumin) or, where the packed cell volume is less than 30%, blood.

Dextran 70 and haemaccel should be avoided in any patient with known drug allergy or bronchospastic tendency. PPF should be used in the albumin-depleted patient. Maximum volume of dextran 70 advised/24 h is 1.5 g dextran/kg BW.

Blood more than 3 days old has a fall in 2,3 DPG content, a consequent shift of the oxyhaemoglobin dissociation curve to the left and a fall in P_{50} (pressure of oxygen in the arterial blood at 50% saturation haemoglobin). In massive haemorrhage blood less than 3 days old is preferable. Other factors which may lower the P_{50} should also be avoided (Table 3.3).

Management of haemorrhagic shock

The commonest cause of acute shock is haemorrhage. If the source is not readily found, consider the following:
1 Any evidence of gastro-intestinal bleeding
   • gastric aspirate, rectal examination
2 Any evidence of intraperitoneal bleeding:
   • pancreatitis
   • trauma
   • ruptured spleen
   • ruptured vascular aneurysm
3 Any evidence of retroperitoneal bleeding:
   • pancreatitis
   • trauma

The severity of shock (percentage of blood volume loss) can be related to clinical findings — the young patient may, however, vasoconstrict and produce few clinical manifestations until the phase of moderate shock. Postural hypotension is, however, always present (Table 3.4).

3.0 Shock

3.3 Changes in circulating blood volume

The general management of haemorrhagic shock is summarized in Table 3.5. The more specific management of gastro-intestinal haemorrhage (Table 4.66, p. 223) and pancreatitis (Table 4.72, p. 228) is summarized elsewhere.

The volume of blood lost can be estimated according to Table 3.4 and in the case of traumatic shock an estimate should also be made according to the extent of injuries (Table 3.6).

When volume is being replaced rapidly, it is essential to estimate sequentially the right atrial pressure (Table 1.2, p. 18) and should the estimated volume lost be replaced (with blood colloid or albumin-containing solution) and the patient remain shocked, a hidden source of haemorrhage or a surgically correctable lesion (ruptured spleen, ruptured aortic aneurysm) should be considered. The ratio of blood to other fluids to be given is summarized in Table 3.7. On occasions it may be necessary to take the patient to theatre for emergency surgery. Under such circumstances the following aspects of patient management are essential:

1 In massive haemorrhage, consider planned intubation and ventilation prior to transfer to theatre.
2 Avoid muscle relaxants if at all possible and avoid potent analgesics unless facilities are available for resuscitation should respiratory depression occur.
3 Check clotting factors, platelets, Hb, PCV, U&E, BG, Astrup, prior to transfer.
4 Any abnormalities in the clotting factors, consult haematology department. Give four packs of FFP prior to transfer and have more packs defrosted for theatre. Platelet count $<60 \times 10^9/l$ give 4-6 packs before theatre, 4-6 packs during operation and consider 4-6 packs postoperatively.
5 Evidence of ARF (Table 2.22, p. 86) give dextrose insulin prior to theatre should Se K be >4.0, and make arrangements for renal dialysis post-operatively. (A peritoneal dialysis catheter or an A-V shunt can be prepared in theatre). Ensure adequate ventilation in theatre and avoid fluid overload.
6 Drips must be placed in the upper part of the body; at least two drips should be running in addition to the RAP line.
7 All fluids given intravenously must be warmed. Place the patient on a warming blanket prior to theatre and whilst on the table, monitor core temperature.
8 Should there be time and facilities available, insert an intra-arterial line (preferably dorsalis pedis) for monitoring of blood pressure (BP) and for blood sampling.

9 Avoid a metabolic alkalosis, hypokalaemia, hyperkalaemia and/or hypoxia. Treat hyperglycaemia with short-acting insulin if BG >12.0 mmol/l.

10 Avoid drugs which may produce myocardial depression.

11 Do not use muscle relaxants until the abdomen is opened. Shock on the operating table in the presence of a high normal RAP may be due to:
   - cardiac factors
   - acute tension pneumothorax

12 Postoperatively do not reverse the anaesthetic but return patient to the ITU ventilated.
   Consider extubation 24 h later, provided:
   - haemodynamic state is stable
   - no chest injury necessitating ventilation
   - $PaO_2 > 9.0$ kPa/(67.5 mmHg) on inspiratory oxygen percentage of >0.35.

3.4 Particular aspects of trauma

Introduction

The management of multiple trauma can be summarized as follows:

1 Preservation of the airway.

2 Ensure adequate ventilation (by intubation and ventilation if necessary).

3 Assessment of the extent of the injuries and appropriate volume replacement (Table 3.5).

4 Appropriate investigative procedures.

5 Surgery either immediately or after period of observation.

6 Continued supportive care.

The management of chest injuries is described on p. 50.

Management of head injuries

A head injury may occur in isolation or be associated with other injuries. It is suggested by some that a CAT (computerized axial tomography) scan should be performed in all patients who have sustained a head injury, but where this is not possible rigorous sequential observation of the patient is essential and should there be deterioration in the level of consciousness, or lateralizing signs develop, a CAT scan is indicated.

3.4 Particular aspects of trauma

Observations should be based on a sequential observation chart (Fig. 3.1). Indications for intubation and ventilation of the head-injured patient are controversial; suggested indications are enumerated in Table 3.8. When ventilation is indicated, sedation should be used which can be lightened rapidly for patient assessment.

Indications for patient transfer to a neurosurgical centre include:
1 Deterioration in the level of consciousness.

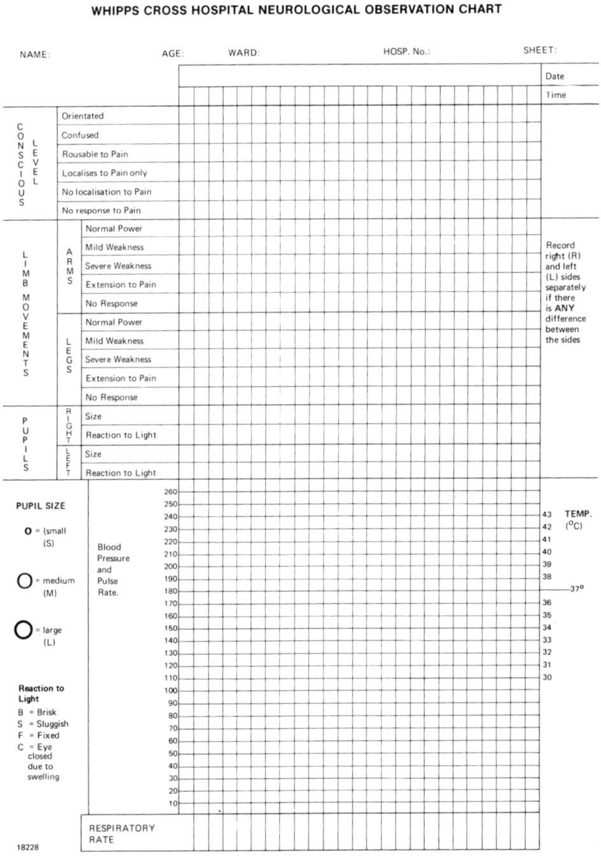
WHIPPS CROSS HOSPITAL NEUROLOGICAL OBSERVATION CHART

NAME: AGE: WARD: HOSP. No.: SHEET:

Date
Time

CONSCIOUS LEVEL
Orientated
Confused
Rousable to Pain
Localises to Pain only
No localisation to Pain
No response to Pain

LIMB MOVEMENTS
ARMS
Normal Power
Mild Weakness
Severe Weakness
Extension to Pain
No Response
LEGS
Normal Power
Mild Weakness
Severe Weakness
Extension to Pain
No Response

Record right (R) and left (L) sides separately if there is ANY difference between the sides

PUPILS
RIGHT
Size
Reaction to Light
LEFT
Size
Reaction to Light

PUPIL SIZE
O = (small (S)
O = medium (M)
O = large (L)

Reaction to Light
B = Brisk
S = Sluggish
F = Fixed
C = Eye closed due to swelling

Blood Pressure and Pulse Rate.
260 250 240 230 220 210 200 190 180 170 160 150 140 130 120 110 100 90 80 70 60 50 40 30 20 10

TEMP. (°C)
43 42 41 40 39 38 37° 36 35 34 33 32 31 30

RESPIRATORY RATE

18228

Fig. 3.1.

3.0 Shock

3.4 Particular aspects of trauma

2 Development of localizing signs.
3 Craniocerebal missile injuries.
4 Compound depressed skull fracture.
5 Closed depressed skull fracture when the depression is greater than the thickness of the skull and where there are focal neurological signs.

The management of head injury is enumerated in Table 3.9.

Management of spinal injuries

Basic principles

Should a spinal injury be suspected, the following principles are of importance:

1 Suspect in all unconscious patients or in a conscious patient who is unable to move legs or arms, or complains of loss of feeling.
2 When suspected—assess the likely nature and extent of injury by history. Rotate the patient *in one piece* to examine the spine and look for discoloration.
3 An early neurological examination is essential.
4 In cervical lesions observe the airway and ventilation. Lesions of C_3 and C_5 are unlikely to survive without respiratory assistance. Autonomic damage may require treatment.
5 Severe spinal injuries are commonly associated with other injuries which may mask the spinal injury (e.g. head injury, chest injury). It is essential that the spinal injury is diagnosed early since incorrect movement may lead to paresis.
6 Skilled nursing care is essential. The skin of the paraplegic below the spinal lesion is very susceptible to trauma.

Management of a cervical injury

This is the injury most commonly encountered in the Intensive Therapy Unit and its management is summarized in Table 3.10.

Management of abdominal injuries

Abdominal injury is likely following trauma if there are fractures of the lower rib cage, or there has been an injury to the abdominal wall.

3.0 Shock

3.4 Particular aspects of trauma

Crushing injuries (e.g. due to a maladjusted seat belt) may produce rupture of a viscus or pancreatitis.

The management of abdominal injuries is summarized in Table 3.11.

Management of burns

The patient with severe burns after initial resuscitation in the Accident and Emergency department should be transferred to the nearest burns unit.

The management of severe burns is described in detail by Davies (1978).

Management of injuries of the genito-urinary tract

Should rupture of the urethra or bladder be suspected, catheterization must not be performed. An urgent high dose IVP (intravenous pyelography) should be arranged after the initial resuscitation. When the IVP suggests a bladder rupture alone, an ascending urethrogram or cystogram may be necessary. Where rupture of the urethra is suspected, a suprapubic cystotomy is generally performed — expert urological advice is essential.

Where GU (genito-urinary) trauma is suspected and laparotomy is indicated, the surgeon must be asked to explore the GU tract.

Renal trauma is generally treated conservatively but a urological opinion is advisable.

Management of electrical and lightning injuries

Electrical injuries
Alternating current (a.c.) is more dangerous than direct current (d.c.) of similar intensity. As the number of cycles is increased in a.c. the danger is decreased, since muscle and nerves are less sensitive to high frequencies. The degree of tissue damage in an electric injury is proportional to the amperage (intensity):

- amps (intensity) = volts (potential difference)/ohms (resistance)
  where amps (intensity) = coulombs/second
  volts (potential difference) = joules/coulomb

High tension injuries and lightning injuries

In these injuries locking to the contact is uncommon and the patient may be thrown away, sustaining multiple injuries.

The lightning stroke is complex; there may be forty successive current peaks of 10 000-200 000 amps with a potential difference of up to 20 million volts.

The urgent complications which may arise following an electrical or lightning injury are enumerated in Table 3.12 and management is summarized in Table 3.13.

3.5 Shock and sepsis

Introduction

Haemodynamic changes found in septic shock are extremely variable, the majority (once circulating blood volume has been replaced) manifest initially with a normal or increased cardiac output and a decreased or normal peripheral vascular resistance. Subsequent changes are so variable that elaborate monitoring may be required in order to apply appropriate haemodynamic support. Patients who present with a low cardiac output have either an inadequate circulating blood volume (common) preceding myocardial dysfunction, or have developed cardiac failure because of inability to keep up with circulating demands (common in the elderly), or because of myocardial depression associated with sepsis.

Few patients if treated appropriately should die within the first 48 h unless diagnosis is made late.

The differential diagnosis is summarized in Table 3.14. Early diagnosis and treatment is essential and where there are signs suggestive of this condition, sepsis must be presumed to be the cause until proven otherwise.

General management

Sequence of treatment is summarized in Table 3.15 and management in Table 3.16.

3.0 Shock

3.5 Shock and sepsis

It is wise to transfer the patient with suspected severe sepsis to an ITU early since the rate of deterioration may be extremely rapid.

A history (if necessary from an observer) is essential, since this may give an indication of the source of sepsis. Other essential aspects of the history are recent drug therapy; preceding evidence of organ failure; contact with an infectious disease; and details of any recent surgery.

Physical examination should be performed, if possible, before the use of drugs which may hide clinical signs (e.g. analgesics). The monitoring systems considered essential in patient management are enumerated in Table 3.17. (The value of these indices is summarized in the table on p. 14).

Monitoring systems may require to be more esoteric if the haemo-dynamic state cannot be adequately evaluated. These systems are enumerated in the Table 3.18. (The value of these indices is summarized in the table on p. 18). On rare occasions other investigations are required and these are listed in Table 3.19.

Sequential management (see Tables 3.15 and 3.16)

Treatment of shock associated with sepsis has been described in detail (Hanson, 1978[2]).

Respiratory control
Hypoxia secondary to intrinsic lung pathology or factors secondary to sepsis leading to a shunt and/or increasing alveolar arterial oxygen gradient is common. Ventilation should be introduced early rather than late because:
1 Hypoxia may produce organ function deterioration.
2 Patient tires easily if hypoxic since hyperventilation is necessary.
3 The critically ill patient is likely to aspirate.
4 Intra-abdominal sepsis requiring surgery is associated with diaphragmatic splinting basal atelectasis and a high incidence of aspiration.

Indications for ventilation include the following:
1 PaO_2 <10.0 kPa/75 mmHg) in a deteriorating patient.
2 Inability to maintain a PaO_2 >9.0 kPa/(67.5 mmHg) with oxygen via a mask.

3 Suggestive evidence of 'shock lung'.
4 Likelihood of pulmonary aspiration (in particular a near-term pregnancy).
5 Patient due for surgery.

Intubation must be performed by a skilled operator with an assistant and good suction facilities available.

Hand ventilation is essential initially since the haemodynamic state may be so unstable that loss of the negative phase associated with artificial ventilation may be followed by a fall in cardiac output (CO).

Should this be suspected, a RAP (right atrial pressure) line should be introduced if at all possible prior to intubation (see below).

In severe hypoxia ventilation/perfusion must be matched in order to achieve adequate oxygenation. This commonly requires the insertion of a thermodilution probe and adjusting circulating volume CO and ventilatory indices in order to achieve optimum ventilation/perfusion (p. 42).

Inspiratory oxygen percentage must be monitored with care and a level of 0.5 or above avoided for >24 h.

PEEP (positive and expiratory pressure) may be necessary when a $PaO_2 > 9.0$ kPa/(67.5 mmHg) cannot be achieved. This must be applied with care because of the common adverse affect on the haemodynamic state (p. 42).

Volume and metabolic control
The majority of patients require restoration of the circulating blood volume based on the RAP and a series of fluid challenges (Fig. 3.2). A low RAP (<4 cm H_2O measured in the mid-axilla with the patient in the horixontal plane) in the presence of shock, is clearly due to depletion of circulating blood volume. A level of 4-14 cm H_2O may be due to hypovolaemia, normovolaemia or when >6 cm H_2O, the patient may have a raised PCWP (pulmonary capillary wedge pressure). At this level in the presence of shock, 200 ml aliquots of appropriate fluid (generally PPF) is infused every 15 min until the RAP rises rapidly and fails to fall, or until the patient's general condition has improved (BP (blood pressure) SP (systolic pressure) >100 mm, improved urine output). A sudden rise in RAP is an indication to stop the infusion since it generally indicates volume overload, and/or inadequate myocardial response to loading (Fig. 3.2).

3.5 Shock and sepsis

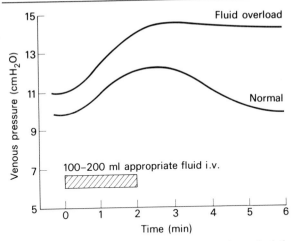

Fig. 3.2. Sequential observations during therapeutic manipulations. The RAP fluid challenge.

Type of fluid to select—a protein-containing solution is preferable since an attempt should be made to maintain the Se albumin 30 g or above and the COP (colloid osmotic pressure) above 20 mmHg. Blood should *not* be used unless the PCV (packed cell volume) is <30%.

Large volumes of crystalloid should be avoided since complicating interstitial oedema is common.

Observe the Se K and where Ca, Mag, PO_4 are likely to be depleted (p. 143) these should also be checked and corrected appropriately.

Hypokalaemia is common when BP and renal perfusion are restored rapidly and may be further lowered with the use of steroids and/or insulin.

BG is commonly normal and rises as the patient improves. A BG >12.0 mmol/l is an indication for insulin.

A metabolic acidosis is common and should not be corrected unless 7.2 or less. With improvement in perfusion and oxygenation pH improves spontaneously. A pH of 7.2 or less which, in spite of bicarbonate replacement, keeps falling is an adverse sign and indicates generally a refractory lactic acidosis (p. 153). Shocked

patients do not tolerate sodium loading and this has to be considered when giving repeated doses of sodium bicarbonate.

The use of steroids is controversial, but evidence to date suggests
they are of value when there has been an inadequate response to
the above measures. 2.0 g methyl prednisolone (30 mg/kg BW) is
given as a bolus and may be repeated on one or two occasions
over the subsequent 24 h should the patient's condition remain
critical.

Should the BP remain low, peripheral perfusion poor and there be
evidence of organ failure in spite of the above measures, circulating volumes must be optimized by fluid loading using the
PCWP, and inotropes are likely to be required. This clinical
picture is commonly seen when CO is inadequate; there may be
associated peripheral vasoconstriction or a low CO state with high
peripheral perfusion.

An indication that myocardial depression is present may be shown
by the response to a fluid challenge (Fig. 3.3). An inappropriately
slow pulse is also commonly present.

The inotropes commonly used are shown in the table on pp. 77
and 78; the inotrope to select is shown in Table 3.20. High doses
of any inotrope should be avoided — a normal BP is not the objec-
tive. The dose should be kept to a minimum being content with
an adequate femoral artery pulse pressure and peripheral perfusion, normal cerebration, a decrease in the metabolic acidosis and
a BP SP of 80 mmHg or more. In these extremely ill patients
acute renal failure (ARF) is common and therefore urine output
may not increase with improved perfusion. Onset of acute atrial
fibrillation is common in the elderly.

Dopamine in high dosage should be avoided since it may produce
an adrenergic effect with increasing SVR (systemic vascular
resistance) — I have never been forced to use a peripheral vasodilator in the presence of a high SVR. Should an agent be considered essential (falling skin temperature, increasing lactic
acidosis), an agent which can be rapidly reversed such as nitroprusside should be considered.

High dose dopamine must be avoided and when the haemodynamic benefit has not been achieved with dopamine,
dopamine/dobutamine combination may prove useful.

3.5 Shock and sepsis

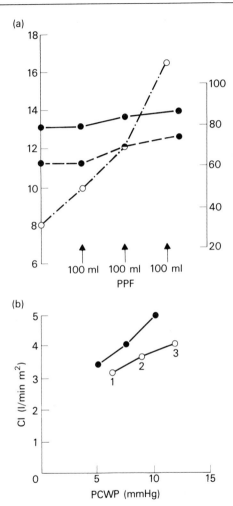

Fig. 3.3. (a) *Myocardial depression during sepsis. Response to volume load.* •---•, *Pulse rate;* •—•, *BP SP;* ○-··-○, *cvp* (*cmH₂O*). (b) *Myocardial depression during sepsis to volume load. 1, 2 and 3 = aliquots of 100 ml PPF infused.* •, *Survivors;* ○, *non-survivors.*

3.0 Shock

3.5 Shock and sepsis

A low CO resistance shock in the author's experience has
a good prognosis. Peripheral vasoconstrictors should not be used
but perfusion improved with an inotrope. Hypotension BP SP
70-80 mmHG is common in this situation and provided cerebration
and oxygenation is adequate, I do not use an inotrope. Renal
failure is likely and should be treated as appropriate (p. 60).

Bacteriological control — bactericidal antibiotics should not be
used until resuscitation is in progress because of the danger of
haemodynamic deterioration following their use (because of the
release of toxin from the bacteria).

The choice depends upon the following conditions (Table 3.21)
and should be made with consultation from the bacteriology
department. Where the patient is critically ill, immunologically
depressed, the source of infection unknown and a resistant
organism suspected, a combination of gentamicin, metronidazole
and piperacillin is probably most suitable. Monitoring of
gentamicin levels is essential.

Where the source of infection is known and the organism suspected to be gram negative, then a combination of cefuroxime
and metronidazole is suitable.

Antibiotic therapy should be as specific as possible and should be
revised after 24 h when bacteriology should be available. Antibiotics alone will *not save* the patient if there is an infective
source amenable to surgery.

DIC (disseminated intravascular coagulation) is common in the
presence of sepsis and can be diagnosed on a series of simple
indices (Table 3.22). Treatment should be considered if the KPTT
(kaolin partial thromboplastin time) or P-T (prothrombin time)
is prolonged greater than $3 \times$ normal and/or platelet count
$<40/10^9/l$ DIC should also be treated with FFP (fresh frozen
plasma) if there is a known coagulation defect and the patient
is due to go to theatre. Treatment of DIC is summarized in
Table 3.23.

Surgery is indicated under the following circumstances:
- a known source of sepsis amenable to surgery
- shock associated with a suspected intraperitoneal source of
  sepsis
- renal infection associated with an obstructive uropathy

3.5 Shock and sepsis

- severe shock—where the source of infection is uncertain but an intra-abdominal cause is possible

It is essential that the patient's condition is optimized prior to surgery, and surgery should be conducted by an experienced surgeon as soon as the haemodynamic state has been stabilized. The procedures to be undertaken pre-, per- and postoperatively are summarized in Tables 3.24-3.26.

Unusual types of shock and sepsis

Certain types of infection require specific therapy in addition to the measures already mentioned.

Anaerobic infections and dermal gangrene
Anaerobic infections can be diagnosed by the analysis of material from the site of infection (Fig. 3.4). Associated diabetes mellitus is common. The majority require major surgical debridement and clostridial infection HBO (hyperbaric oxygen) therapy (Hanson, 1978[3]) before and after surgery.

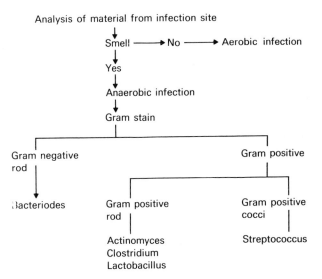

Fig. 3.4. Diagnosis of anaerobic infections.

3.0 Shock

3.5 Shock and sepsis

Acute dermal gangrene includes necrotizing fasciitis and progressive bacterial gangrene.

Necrotizing fasciitis is a rapidly progressive necrotizing process which affects the subcutaneous fat, superficial fascia and upper surface of the deep fascia. The condition commonly follows abdominal surgery (6-31 days later) and is associated with extreme toxaemia. Treatment includes resuscitation and major surgical debridement.

Progressive bacterial gangrene commonly involves the perineum — the whole thickness of the skin is involved and a little subcutaneous tissue. The patient may be toxic but rarely as ill as in necrotizing fasciitis. Treatment includes resuscitation, surgery and debridement. Epithelialization is generally rapid.

Acute toxic shock syndrome (TSS)
This condition predominantly affects healthy young women. A higher percentage develop during menstruation and are associated with the use of tampons, approximately 13% are *not* associated with menstruation. The organism is a Staphylococcus of predominantly phage group 1, lysed by phage 29 and resistant only to penicillin. It is characterized by the presence of a staphylococcal enterotoxin F. The major clinical signs are fever, hypotension (often associated with organ failure) and an erythematous rash associated with desquamation. Diagnosis is essential so that in addition to resuscitation, an anti-staphylococcal antibiotic is used (Editorial, 1982).

Tetanus
Tetanus is a condition produced by the release of tetanus toxin from the lysed spores of *C. tetani.* The bacteria are strict anaerobes. The condition is rare in the UK, only fifteen cases (two fatal) being notified in 1978. Most of the cases in the UK have been in elderly gardeners, agricultural workers and young sportsmen.

The condition must be diagnosed early since misdiagnosis may lead to death from pulmonary aspiration.

The incubation period — the interval between the wounding and the onset of the first spasm — varies between 3-21 days. A long interval is no guarantee of a mild attack. The period of onset (the interval between the first symptom and first spasm) is of prognostic significance — the shorter the interval the more severe the attack.

When tetanus is suspected, other conditions producing similar symptoms must be excluded (Table 3.27). If the diagnosis is in doubt, admit to the ITU and observe.

Once tetanus is diagnosed, the illness should be classified and treatment based on classification (Table 3.28).

Treatment. The following steps should be taken:

1 Excise wound (if present) and pack with hydrogen peroxide.
2 Benzylpenicillin 1 MU i.m. or i.v. 6-hourly for 7 days.
3 Observe for superinfection.
4 Tetanus antitoxin (Humotet) 30 iu/kg i.m.
5 Give first dose of antitoxin at the same time.

The patient may move from one grade to the next so careful observation is necessary. Management is summarized below:

Grade 1
- pulmonary aspiration is unlikely
- sedate with diazepam
- pass a Ryles tube, give antacids and observe ventilation
- do not feed orally for at least 3 days, give fluids intravenously during this period
- once symptons resolved (generally after a few days) and there has been no deterioration, start light oral diet and discharge to wards.

Grade 2
- early tracheostomy
- Ryles tube antacids
- sedate with diazepam
- observe tidal volume, and respiratory rate
- use opiates if there is pain from spasms or wound site

Grade 3
- early tracheostomy
- Ryles tube antacids
- spasms uncontrolled with diazepam, danger of respiratory depression
- use a muscle relaxant: curare — if there is tachycardia hypertension; pancuronium — if there is bradycardia hypotension
- ensure adequate sedation, tranquillization and analgesia

- use a combination of diazepam or lorazepam: chlorpromazine; opiates

Discuss drug therapy with someone who has had experience in treating tetanus—it is essential that relaxation is full and that the patient is well sedated and tranquillized so that on recovery there is no memory of the event.

After 2 weeks, muscle relaxants are stopped and sedatives tailed off. Stiffness rarely persists for more than 3 weeks.

Autonomic dysfunction
This develops 1-4 days after neuromuscular blockade and lasts up to 10 days.

Management is difficult since activity is very variable, consisting of fluctuating hypertension, tachycardia and cardiac arrhythmias. Episodes of hypotension, bradycardia and occasionally asystole. Best to use drugs intravenously which can be rapidly withdrawn and have a relatively short duration of activity.

Sympathetic overactivity:
1 Sedate the patient heavily.
2 Use intravenous practolol for tachycardia >140/min. Use intravenous labetolol if associated with hypertension DP (diastolic pressure >110.
3 Bradycardia precipitated by stimulation, e.g. tracheostomy suction, give intravenous atropine prior to procedure.
4 Bradycardia and hypotension—volume top-up if RAP <4 cm H_2O and intravenous isoprenaline as an infusion titrated until pulse rate >70/min.
5 Asystole—the heart will often start with a blow on the sternum. Give intracardiac adrenaline if necessary or if followed by bradycardia, isoprenaline infusion.

General management. The following points should be noted:
1 It is essential to ensure normal oxygenation and $PaCO_2$.
2 Superinfection is common.
3 Nitrogen losses are high; feeding via a Ryles tube is preferable but ileus is common—then intravenous nutrition is necessary.
4 Careful fluid and metabolic balance is essential since in severe tetanus with autonomic dysfunction, compensation is inadequate for hypovolaemia or fluid overload.
5 Prophylactic heparin and antacids are essential.

3.0 Shock

3.5 Shock and sepsis

Pneumonia
The patient may be admitted to the ITU with severe pneumonia, or it may arise whilst the patient is being treated in the ITU.

Pneumonia may present with shock associated with sepsis, but has the additional problem that, when severe, ARDS makes resuscitation difficult.

The prognosis of shock and extensive pneumonia is poor.

The principles of resuscitation from shock (Table 3.16) and treatment as for ARDS (p. 45) still apply.

Nature of shock—a high percentage of patients present with a high CO and low SVR. Inotropes should not be used unless SP is sufficiently low to produce oliguria and/or decrease pulmonary perfusion.

Inotropes—use with *great care*, may increase the intrapulmonary shunt. Should shunt increase and PaO_2 fall, give supportive care for renal failure and withdraw inotropes. (Dosage of dopamine 1-2 μg/kg may be sufficient to maintain renal perfusion.)

Adjustment of CO in relation to ventilation is essential—high levels of PEEP should be avoided (increasing the incidence of pneumothorax).

The organisms responsible are listed in Table 3.29.

Gram stain of the tracheal aspirate (after intubation of the trachea) is essential and will often give the diagnosis, but where there are no organisms present, Legionella, mycoplasma, or one of the unusual pneumonias found in the immunocompromised host, should be suspected.

Appropriate tests must be taken to confirm the diagnosis of Rickettsial, *chlamydia psittaci*, Legionella, mycoplasma and Cytomegalovirus infections.

Where the gram stain is negative, erythromycin must be added to the antibiotic regimen.

Additional features may make one suspect certain types of pneumonia (Table 3.30).

Where the diagnosis is in doubt, paraquat intoxication, pulmonary aspiration, or ARDS due to a non-pulmonary cause, must be excluded.

Table 3.1. Causes of shock due to fluid overload in the absence of known myocardial disease

---

Acute water intoxication
Acute sodium/water overload
Moderate sodium/water overload in the presence of oliguria
Moderate sodium/water overload in the presence of:
   myocardial depressant drugs
   steroid therapy
   peripheral vasoconstrictors
Over-infusion with an oncotic agent:
   mannitol
   dextrans
Acute hyperosmolar state

Table 3.2. Shock due to a decrease in circulating blood volume

---

Fluid losses
   Stomach
   Biliary tract and pancreas
   Bowel
   Renal—osmotic diuresis
         post-obstructive diuresis
         polyuric renal failure
   Diabetes insipidus
   Skin loss—sweating
   Pulmonary loss—hyperventilation (rare)
   Plasma loss due to destruction of the skin—burns
                      infection
                      major debridement
                      skin disorders e.g.
                        exfoliative
                        dermatitis
   Lack of fluid replacement
   Fluid translocation—increased capillary permeability
             e.g. severe shock.
             peripheral vasodilatation
             e.g. shock and sepsis, epidural blockade
   Renal dialysis
   Blood loss—haemorrhage

3.6 Tables

Table 3.3. Factors which may lower P_{50}

Fall in central body temperature.

Metabolic alkalosis

Old blood ⎫
Phosphate deficiency ⎭ fall in RBC 2,3 DPG

Table 3.4. Haemorrhagic shock. Classification in relation to clinical criteria and percentage of total blood volume lost

Classification	Blood loss as a percentage of total blood volume	Blood pressure (mmHg)	Symptoms and signs
Compensated pre-shock	10-15	Normal	Palpitations Dizziness Tachycardia
Mild	15-30	Slight fall	Palpitations Thirst Tachycardia Weakness Sweating
Moderate	30-35	70-80	Restlessness Pallor Oliguria
Severe	35-40	50-70	Pallor Cyanosis Collapse
Profound	40-50	50	Collapse Air hunger Anuria

Estimated blood volume in healthy non-pregnant individuals as a percentage of body weight:

Body build	Normal	Obese	Thin	Muscular
Blood volume % of body weight	6.5	5.5	6.0	7.0

Table 3.5. Summary of treatment of haemorrhagic shock

Fluids

Compensated pre-shock
(10-15% of blood
volume lost)

Set up drip
Crossmatch

Mild shock
(15-30% of blood
volume lost)

Replace blood volume with
dextran 70, haemaccel or normal
saline

Moderate shock
(30-35% of blood
volume lost)

Replace initially with dextran 70
(max. 1.5 g/kg BW/24 h),
haemaccel or normal saline. Give
blood after full crossmatch, ratio
of blood to other fluid 1:2.
Warm the blood. Filter if more
than 48 h old

Severe shock
(35-40% of blood
volume lost)

At least 2 drips running. Insert a
RAP line. Restore blood volume
as quickly as possible; blood can
generally be partially cross-
matched. Ratio of blood to other
fluid 1:1. Warm the blood. Filter
if blood more than 48 h old

Profound shock
(greater than 40% of
volume lost)

Observe the airway, give oxygen.
Consider intubation. Ratio of
blood to other fluid 1:1 until
80% or more of the blood
volume lost. Under such circumstances give emergency ABO
and rhesus-specific blood. Ratio
blood to other fluid 2:1. Give
50% of blood requirement as
blood stored less than 2 days.
Packed cells should not be used.
Maintain Hct around 30%. Use
PPF as non-haemoglobin containing fluid of choice. Insert
RAP line

Catheterize. Monitor ECG, electrolyte, acid-base status and coagulation profile. Give three packets of FFP for every 4000 ml of blood infused.

Drugs

Sodium bicarbonate: to be given if base deficit >10 and/or pH 7.1 or less. (Aliquots of 50 mmol HCO_3^- or less.)

Mannitol: give 0.2 g/kg BW over 2-3 min if RAP* >4 cm H_2O
BP SP >90 mm/hg and urine output <40 ml/h
Check U/P osmolality ratio before giving mannitol

Potassium chloride: if Se K 3.5 mmol or less, give cautiously in patients with suspected renal failure

Digitalis: consider in patients with a preceding history of heart failure

Insulin: consider if BG >12 mmol/l

Oxygen: if PaO_2 <9.3 kPa (70 mmHg) on oxygen via a face mask, intubate and ventilate

Do not use vasoconstrictors

Do not use muscle relaxants in patients with severe haemorrhagic shock due to an intra-abdominal bleed until blood volume replacement is adequate and the peritoneum has been incised

Should the patient's condition remain serious, in spite of the above measures:
Re-evaluate the respiratory status
Search for obscure sources of bleeding
Consider haemorrhage complicated by sepsis
Assess cardiac function
Exclude a bleeding diathesis

---

*Normal level may be higher than this in patients with preceding high airway pressures or pulmonary hypertension and may be raised acutely because of non-cardiac pulmonary oedema. Under such circumstances this level would not reflect an adequate left ventricular filling pressure and PCWP. Monitoring should be considered (p. 19).

3.6 Tables

Table 3.6. Approximate volume of blood lost from various sites of injury in a 70 kg male (blood volume 5.0) (modified from London, 1968)

Site of injury	Extent of injury and approximate volume of blood required (ml) and expressed as a percentage of blood volume (5.0 l)			
	Moderate	Total blood volume (%)	Severe	Total blood volume (%)
Arm and forearm	400	8	1200	24
Foot and ankle	400	8	800	16
Leg	800	16	1800	36
Thigh	1200	24	2500	50
Pelvis	1200	24	5000	100
Abdomen	1200	24	5000	100
Chest	1200	24	5000	100

Table 3.7. Haemorrhagic shock. Ratio of blood to other fluid

Estimated total volume of blood loss as a percentage of total blood volume	Therapeutic regime
<30	Blood not required. (use PPF if Se albumin likely to be low)
30-80	Ratio of blood to other fluid, 1:1
>80	Idem. 2:1
	50% should preferably be blood stored less than 3 days. If not, clotting factor replacement essential

Table 3.8. Indications for ventilation in severe head injury

Associated serious pulmonary pathology
Control of epilepsy
Acute reduction in ICP
Transfer of a serious head injury to a neurological unit where
airway control is in doubt

Table 3.9. Management of head injury

1   Maintain the airway
2   Restore metabolic and fluid balance
    Insert a RAP line and maintain at 2-6 cm H_2O; *do not*
    overload.
3   Ventilate according to Table 3.8.
    In head injury it is advisable to hyperventilate, maintain a
    PaO_2 10-12 kPa (75-90 mmHg) and $PaCO_2$ 3.7-4.0 kPa.
    (28-30 mmHg)
4   Careful neurological assessment of associated injuries
    Start the head injury observation chart (see figure on p. 99)
5   Skull X-ray and other X-rays if necessary
    Consider a CAT scan
6   Transfer patient to a neurosurgical unit according to p. 99
7   Dexamethasone is of controversial value
8   Antacids or cimetidine
9   Mannitol in our practice is reserved for patients with evidence
    of a rapid onset rise in ICP and is used in conjunction with
    hyperventilation
    Mannitol 25% give 2.0 g/kg BW over 30 min and repeat
    6-hourly. *Do not* give if fluid overload present
    Observe Se K after its use
10 Anticonvulsants, do not give routinely
    Convulsions use phenytoin i.v.
11 Analgesics—do not use long-acting opiates. Use dihydro-
    codeine tartrate 30-60 mg titrated intravenously. When
    ventilated, coughing and straining must be prevented; the
    means of sedation is controversial

3.6 Tables

Table 3.10. Management of cervical fractures

1 2-3 kg of traction should be applied to the head as soon as possible

 Advice from the orthopaedic team is essential since positioning is important and depends upon the type of fracture

2 Nurse on a firm flat bed and alter pressure points every 2 h

 The type of bed varies from one unit to another

3 Observe central body temperature—keep well covered, use a space blanket and maintain room temperature at 20°C

4 Pain relief and anxiety relief may require dihydrocodeine and diazepam

 Titrate intravenously with care, give the minimum and observe the airway and respiratory excursion

5 Ventilation. Respiratory difficulties are usual for the first 24 h

 Ventilation may be required because of an associated chest injury

 Lesion below C_5, ventilation is generally adequate but may deteriorate because of oedema. Ventilation may be adequate during the day but may develop respiratory arrest at night

 C_3 C_4 C_5 lesions rarely survive without respiratory assistance

 C_1 C_2 lesions may have little respiratory upset

6 Bowel. Abdominal distension and ileus is common. Insert a Ryles tube and leave on continuous drainage. Use antacids. Nurse in slight head-up foot-down tilt—observe for pulmonary aspiration

7 Haemodynamic state. Hypotension due to autonomic damage may last for several days and is complicated commonly by bradycardia, particularly after tracheal suction

 Insert a RAP line, ensure adequate circulating volume; if hypotension sufficiently severe to produce oliguria, nurse in slight head down position

 On rare occasions tracheal suction may be complicated by cardiac arrest. Severe bradycardia will respond to i.v. atropine which should on occasions be used routinely prior to tracheal suction

8 Metabolic state. Intravenous feeding may be necessary for up to 1 week because of ileus

9 Bladder. Insert bladder catheter and put on continuous drainage

 Observe for oliguria and urinary infection

3.0 Shock

3.6 Tables

10 Drugs
   Analgesia and sedation   Dihydrocodeine
                            diazepam or lorazepam
   Anti-oedema agents   Consider dexamethasone
                            8 mg i.v. 4-hourly for 3 days
   Antacids
11 Atlas axis fractures commonly associated with head and
   facial injuries
   Skull traction is required. Tracheostomize early

Table 3.11. Management of suspected abdominal injury

1 Careful patient assessment of sites of trauma
2 Observe the airway, intubate and ventilate if necessary
3 Replace volume, insert a RAP line and observe sequentially
4 Pass a Ryles tube and drain the stomach
5 Measure abdominal girth, if fluid suspected, 4 quadrant tap
6 Where intra-abdominal bleeding may develop (e.g. from a
   ruptured spleen or liver), consider insertion of a peritoneal
   dialysis catheter and lavage. (The author finds it more
   reliable to observe fluid balance, RAP and 4 quadrant tap if
   necessary.) Abdominal ultrasound is often helpful
7 *Check* straight X-ray of abdomen, supine and erect; chest
   X-ray and if necessary X-ray of lumbar spine
8 Laparotomy is indicated when:
   There is evidence of concealed haemorrhage (RAP keeps
   falling after volume top-up for no apparent reason)
   There is free gas in the peritoneal cavity
   Presence of abdominal rigidity
   Increasing abdominal distension where the cause is unlikely
   to be due to retroperitoneal haematoma formation alone
   In all patients where penetrating injury of the peritoneum is
   suspected

Table 3.12. Complications which may arise following an electrical or lightning injury

Cardiac	Ventricular fibrillation
	Cardiac dysrhythmias including bradyarrhythmias
Respiratory	Respiratory arrest

continued

Table 3.12—*continued*

	Oral and nasal burns producing oedema and airway obstruction Pulmonary aspiration Pulmonary contusion
CNS	Loss of consciousness—respiratory arrest Convulsions Cerebral oedema Subarachnoid or intracerebral haemorrhage
Bone	Fractures Joint dislocations Lesions of the spine producing quadraplegia, paraplegia
Bowel	Ileus—vomiting and fluid loss Gastric haemorrhage
Deep tissues	Muscle necrosis and soft tissue oedema—producing loss of intravascular volume
Skin	Second and third degree burns with fluid loss
Blood vessels	Vessel occlusion with subsequent tissue and muscle necrosis
Kidneys	Tubular necrosis—acute renal failure
Metabolic	Metabolic acidosis Fluid volume depletion with attendant metabolic deficits Exposure hypothermia

Table 3.13. Management of electrical or lightning injuries

1　Establish routine resuscitative procedures
2　Detect if at all possible the inflow and exit sites, and the current of injury, giving an indication of tissue damage which may have occurred (see table 3.12)

Particular aspects of resuscitation and subsequent management

1　Cardiac:
　　Cardiac asystole is common and will often respond to intracardiac adrenaline. Persistent ventricular dysrhythmias—use

lignocaine. Persistent supraventricular dysrhythmias — use practolol. Give intermittent bolus injections titrating intravenously the minimum amount of drug required to produce a therapeutic effect.

2 Respiratory:
Respiratory arrest — ventilate
Lung contusion — ventilate if severe
Pulmonary aspiration — ventilate
Rib fractures — ventilate if patient hypoxic, otherwise appropriate analgesic

3 Metabolic:
Insert a RAP line, restore blood volume preferably with PPF
Correct metabolic abnormalities
Observe for renal failure and treat accordingly (p. 60)

4 Hypothermia. Rewarm slowly (p. 140)

5 Skin. Estimate extent of burns and replace volume accordingly (Davies, 1978).

6 Central nervous system (CNS). Prolonged arrest, fixed dilated pupils, *do not* assume brain stem death
Give optimum treatment for cerebral oedema including ventilation ($PaCO_2$ 3.7-4.0 kPa [28-30 mmHg]) and dexamethasone 10 mg i.v. 5 hr and 4 mg 6-hourly
Focal signs — CAT scan and neurosurgery if necessary

7 Gastro-intestinal:
Insert Ryles tube and drain stomach contents
Regular antacid therapy
Prolonged ileus is usual — intravenous nutrition often indicated
Observe for:
  onset of pancreatitis
  perforation
  bowel infarction
  gastric haemorrhage
Elicit source of haemorrhage — gastroscopy
If haemorrhage due to stress erosions — start intravenous cimetidine
Haemorrhage refractory and not related to clotting factor deficit — operate

8 Haematological:
Observe clotting factors. DIC may develop following a prolonged cardiac arrest

9 Sepsis:
Secondary infection is common, prophylactic antibiotics not indicated.

continued

Table 3.13— *continued*

10 Surgery may be indicated for:
    Treatment of burns
    Correction of joint injuries or fractures
    Treatment of bowel perforation
                    resection of infarcted bowel
                    gastric haemorrhage

Table 3.14. Differential diagnosis of shock and infection

Early signs	Alternative diagnosis
Pyrexia (occasionally absent)	Myocardial failure
Sweating	Pulmonary embolism
Restlessness	Amniotic fluid embolism
Some confusion	Adverse drug reaction
Tachypnoea	Incompatible blood transfusion
Tachycardia 90-110/min	Transfusion of old blood
Slight fall in BP 80-100 mmHg systolic pressure	Blood volume loss in the absence of septicaemia
Mild jaundice	
Deterioration during anaesthesia or failure to regain consciousness after an anaesthetic	

Late signs	
Coma	Cerebral catastrophe
Tachypnoea often associated with central cyanosis	Myocardial failure
Cold pale extremities with peripheral cyanosis	Pulmonary ⎰ aspiration / thrombotic embolism / amniotic fluid embolism
Skin cold and clammy	
Tachycardia >110/min	Hepatocellular failure
Hypotension <80 mmHg	Blood volume loss in the absence of septicaemia
Moderate jaundice	
Oliguria	
Coagulation abnormalities	

Table 3.15. Sequence of treatment for shock associated with sepsis

1 Respiratory control
2 Volume and metabolic control
3 Additional therapy for shock non-responsive to the above measures
4 Bacteriological control
5 Hyperbaric oxygen
6 Supportive care for organ failure
7 Haematological control
8 Surgery

Table 3.16. Summary of management of shock associated with sepsis

1 Assess adequacy of ventilation. Give oxygen, maintain PaO_2 at 10 kPa (75 mmHg) or above, ventilate if necessary
2 Assess electrolyte, BG and acid base status. Insert a CVP line, restore circulating blood volume and if possible correct metabolic imbalance. Should pH be 7.2 or less, consider bicarbonate 50 mmol i.v. Recheck pH 1 h later
3 Should there be a poor response to (2) give methylprednisolone 2.0 g i.v.
4 Should condition remain critical, consider monitoring PCWP and cardiac output and the use of drugs affecting cardiac function (see table on p. 77)
5 Take blood and other cultures and start appropriate antibiotic therapy. Give antibiotics intravenously
6 In the presence of possible Clostridial sepsis, consider the use of hyperbaric oxygen
7 Measure the U/P osmolality ratio. Insert a bladder catheter and measure urine output. If urine output <40 ml/h and less than 50 h have elapsed from the onset of oliguria and the U/P ratio is less than 2.0, give up to three doses of mannitol (0.2 g/kg body weight) i.v. over 2-3 min at 2-hourly intervals until the urine is at least 50 ml/h
8 Should there be no increase in urine volume and renal failure confirmed, establish the conservative regime for ARF. Assess the appropriate time for dialysis. Reassess the drug dosage in the light of impaired renal function (see p. 20)

continued

Table 3.16— *continued*

9 Assess the haematological status, including evidence of intravascular haemolysis, hypercoagulation or hypo-coagulation. Treat appropriately
10 Consider surgery

Table 3.17. Monitoring systems essential for management of the patient with shock and infection

Pulse rate
Pulse pressure
BP
ECG oscilloscope trace
Central and skin temperatures
Fluid balance. U/P osmolality ratio
BU. Electrolytes, blood gases, acid base state. BG
Respiratory rate
Hb. Hct. WBC and diff. Coagulation indices, platelets
RAP

Table 3.18. More esoteric monitoring systems and derived indices which may be required if the systems in the table above are inadequate in evaluation of the haemodynamic state and/or are essential for therapy

Pulmonary capillary wedge pressure
Cardiac output
Peripheral vascular resistance
Pulmonary compliance
Serum albumin. Colloid oncotic pressure

3.0 Shock

Table 3.19. Shock and sepsis: Investigations required on rare occasions

Haemoglobin molecule analysis

Other indices for haemolysis:
  G- 6-phosphate dehydrogenase
  haptoglobin

Serum folate

Se calcium, magnesium, inorganic phosphate

Serum amylase

LFT's

Australia antigen

Table 3.20. Shock and sepsis: use of inotropes

Haemodynamic state	Inotrope of choice

Cardiac dysrhythmia + CO ↓
  Atrial fibrillation
  Atrial flutter
	Digoxin

Pulse rate <110/min CO ↓ SVR ↑	Isoprenaline
Pulse rate >110/min	Low dose dopamine (<4 μg/kg BW/min) CO still ↓ add dobutamine
CO ↓ SVR ↓	Optimize PCWP with PPF Dopamine up to 6 μg/kg BW/min CO still ↓ add dobutamine
CO ↓ SVR ↑	Low dose dopamine CO still ↓ add dobutamine Evidence of increasing lactic acidosis consider nitroprusside or isosorbide dinitrate (like isoprenaline these agents may increase pulse rate but rarely produce dysrrhythmias)

Table 3.21. Factors affecting antibiotic choice

Patient's preceding condition:
  on immunosuppressives
  diabetic
  anaemic
  already receiving antibiotics
  on long-term steroids

Source of infection $\begin{cases} \text{in hospital} \\ \text{outside hospital} \end{cases}$

Site of infection $\begin{cases} \text{known} \begin{cases} \text{can be surgically drained} \\ \text{not amenable to surgery} \end{cases} \\ \text{unknown} \end{cases}$

Likely organism $\begin{cases} \text{known} \\ \text{unknown} \end{cases}$

Table 3.22. Baseline coagulation studies and changes secondary to transfusion of old blood and DIC

Coagulation test	Normal (non-pregnant) adult	Massive Transfusion	DIC
Platelets	$140\text{-}440 \times 10^9/l$	↓	↓
Prothrombin time	Control ±2.0 sec	↑	↑
KPTT	Control ±7.0 sec	↑	↑
Thrombin time	Control ±2.0 sec	N	↑
Fibrinogen level	160-415 mg/dl	N	↓
or Fibrinogen titre	1/64-1/128	N	< 1/64

Table 3.23. Treatment of DIC

1 Coagulation indices consistent with DIC + cause potentially reversible (e.g. sepsis) and indices $<3\times$ prolonged. Sequential observation. Treat the cause
2 Coagulation indices consistent with DIC and patient due to go to theatre. Give four packets of FFP pre-op. and four packets post-operation
   Platelet count $<60\times10^9/dl$ give platelets — consult haematologist
3 Cause not readily reversible and/or indices $>3\times$ prolonged. Replace labile factors with FFP (one packet of FFP raises the fibrinogen level by approx. 25 mg/100 ml in a 70 kg patient). Do not give platelets unless $<40\times10^9 dl$. Should the fibrogen level (or titre) not rise after four packs of FFP, consider heparin
   Platelet count $<40\times10^9/dl$ in the presence of purpura, or $<60\times10^9/dl$ with adequate clotting factors, give platelets (six to eight packs)
4 Use heparin in all cases where clotting factors repeatedly deteriorate in spite of factor replacement
5 Heparin therapy. 50-100 units/kg BW as a bolus, then 10-15 units/kg BW hourly as a continuous infusion
   Use half recommended dosage if platelets $<100\times10^9/dl$. Monitor clotting factors, reduce dosage of heparin if after therapy TT prolonged >40 S
   Tranexamic acid must *not* be used

Table 3.24. Shock and sepsis. Preparation for operation

Restore circulating blood volume

Correct metabolic imbalance

Correct pulmonary failure

Correct any haematological abnormality

Consider hyperbaric oxygen in the presence of Clostridial sepsis

Check renal function and treat accordingly

Table 3.25. Shock and sepsis. Peroperative management

ECG monitor. Warming blanket

Monitor skin and core temperature if possible

Volume replacement efficient and appropriate

Operative procedure thorough, performed by an experienced surgeon

Intraperitoneal sepsis, consider postoperative lavage

Adequate drainage essential

Renal failure prepare for dialysis

Take blood and other cultures for bacteriology

Table 3.26. Shock and sepsis. Postoperative management

Ventilate postoperatively

Observe for bleeding diathesis

Observe renal function

Observe core temperature

Observe and maintain metabolic balance

Continue hyperbaric oxygen in the presence of Clostridial sepsis or extensive skin debridement with an increased danger of superinfection

Table 3.27. Differential diagnosis of tetanus

Factors causing trismus
  tonsillitis
  dental abscess
  problems relating to the tempero mandibular joint
  hysteria
Muscle spasm
  phenothiazine drugs (rapidly reversed with benztropine mesylate)

Table 3.28. Classification of tetanus according to period of onset (first symptom to first spasm)

Classification	Period of onset in days	Clinical features
Mild (Grade 1)	3-10 days	Mild to moderate trismus and general spasticity Little or no dysphagia No respiratory embarrassment
Moderate (Grade 2)	2-5 days	Moderate trismus and spasticity Some dysphagia and respiratory embarrassment Fleeting spasms
Severe (Grade 3A)	Generally <2 days	Severe trismus. Generalized spasticity and prolonged spasm Dysphagia
Very severe (Grade 3B)		Respiratory embarrassment Evidence of autonomic dysfunction

Table 3.29. Organisms responsible for producing severe pneumonia

Previously healthy individual
  Streptococcus pneumoniae
  Mycoplasma pneumoniae
  Legionella pneumophilia
  Staphylococcus aureus
  H. influenzae
Less commonly
  Klebsiella pneumoniae
  Chlamydia psittaci (psittacosis)
  Coxiella burnetti (Q fever)
  Mycobacterium tuberculosis

continued

Table 3.29—*continued*

The immunocompromised patient
Infection may occur with any of the above but also:
   Pseudomonas sp.
   Proteus sp.
   Anaerobic organisms
   Escherichia coli
   Cytomegalovirus   { *Pneumocystis carinii*
   Fungi and protozoa   { *Aspergillus fumigatus*

Table 3.30. Additional features giving a guide to the organism responsible for producing pneumonia

Previously healthy patient or Immunocompromised patient	See Table 3.29
Lobar involvement	*Streptococcus pneumoniae*
Multiple lung abscesses	*Staphylococcus aureus*
Upper lobe involvement and abscess formation Sputum often viscid jelly-like, often blood stained	*Klebsiella pneumoniae*
Systemic features—diarrhoea confusion Multiple organ failure Hepatomegaly Muscle weakness	*Legionella pneumophilia*
Haemolyte anaemia Cold agglutinins Erythema multiforme	*Mycoplasma pneumoniae*
Occupation Contact with cows and sheep	*Coxiella burnetti*
Contact with birds Hepatosplenomegaly	*Chlamydia psittaci*

3.0 Shock

3.6 Tables

Extensive necrotizing
 pneumonia
Immunocompromised host } *Aspergillus fumigatus*

3.7 References

Davies J. W. L. (1978) The management of the critically ill patient
with severe burns. In *Medical Management of the Critically Ill
Patient* (Ed. by G. C. Hanson & P. L. Wright), p. 443.
Academic Press, London.

Editorial (1982) Toxic shock syndrome: some questions remain.
Brit. Med. J. **284**, 1585.

Hanson G. C. (1978)[1] Shock. Introduction and pathophysiology.
In *Medical Management of the Critically Ill Patient* (Ed. by
G. C. Hanson & P. L. Wright), p. 293. Academic Press,
London.

Hanson G. C. (1978)[2] Shock and infection. In *Medical Management of the Critically Ill Patient* (Ed. by G. C. Hanson &
P. L. Wright), p. 355. Academic Press, London.

Hanson G. C. (1978)[3] The management of gas forming and
anaerobic infections and dermal gangrene. In *Medical
Management of the Critically Ill Patient* (Ed. by G. C. Hanson
& P. L. Wright), p. 49. Academic Press, London.

Hauser C. J., Shoemaker W. C., Turpin I., & Goldberg S. J.
(1980) Oxygen transport responses to colloids and crystalloids
in critically ill surgical patients. *Surg. Gynecol. Obstet.* **150**, 811.

London P. S. (1968) Traumatic shock. *Brit. J. Hosp. Med.* **1**
(3), 312.

3.0 Shock

Notes

3.0 Shock

Notes

4.0 Specific problems

4.1 Disorders in body temperature, 139
Introduction
Hypothermia
Hyperthermia

4.2 Management of acute metabolic disorders, 143
Metabolic response to stress
Management of acute disorders in water and sodium balance
Acute disorders in potassium balance
Disorders of calcium and magnesium balance
Phosphate depletion
Acute disorders of acid base balance
Disorders of uric acid metabolism
Acute disorders of porphyrin metabolism
The hyperosmolar states

4.3 Management of endocrine crises, 158
The thyroid gland
The adrenal gland
Pituitary gland and hypothalamus

4.4 Management of acute disorders of the nervous system
(other than head injury), **160**
Purulent meningitis
Status epilepticus
Acute polyneuropathies
Myasthenia gravis
Brain stem death

4.5 Management of gastro-intestinal emergencies, 163
Massive gastro-intestinal haemorrhage
Inflammatory bowel disease
Acute severe pancreatitis

4.6 Treatment of poisoning, 164
Introduction
General treatment
Particular aspects of management of the more common poisonings
Specific management

4.7 Tables, 173

4.8 References, 235

4.0 Specific problems

4.1 Disorders in body temperature

4.1 Disorders in body temperature

Introduction

Normal body temperature (core) is around $37 \pm 1°C$. A core temperature $<35°C$ is by definition hypothermia. All patients with a core temperature $<30°C$ should be considered seriously ill. Survival is rarely possible at $<24°C$.

There is no clear definition for hyperthermia, however. For instance, in heat stroke the temperature may range from 38-43.8°C depending upon the time interval between onset of symptoms and initial reading of the temperature. Heat damage to tissues occurs at 42°C and survival is unlikely if the core temperature is $>41.2°C$ for a prolonged period.

Hypothermia

Divided into primary hypothermia, acute or chronic, and secondary hypothermia — hypothermia secondary to another disease process.

Clinical features of acute hypothermia
- $<35°C$ dysarthria, disorientation
- $<33°C$ drowsiness, confusion
- $<30°C$ coma, muscle hypertonicity
- $<28°C$ pupillary reflexes absent, muscle flaccidity

Clinical features of chronic hypothermia
Clinical features develop at a temperature 2-3°C lower than in acute hypothermia.

Cardiac changes
- $<35°C$ tachycardia → bradycardia with prolongation of systole
- $<27.2°C$ atrial fibrillation
- $<28°C$ ventricular fibrillation, most commonly if patient disturbed

Haematological changes
Increased haematocrit (due to polyuria)
Oxyhaemoglobin dissociation curve shifted to the left. PaO_2 in solution increases
Oxygen consumption falls
Predisposition to DIC

4.0   Specific problems

4.1   Disorders in body temperature

Respiratory changes
Slowing of respiratory rate. Correction of $PaCO_2$ (arterial carbon dioxide pressure) and pH for body temperature is important and should be requested from the laboratory.

Metabolic changes
Blood glucose (BG)↑; free fatty acids ↑; cortisol ↑

Treatment
Secondary hypothermia treated similarly to primary hypothermia but the underlying disorder may require treatment, e.g. drug over-dose, alcoholism, hypothyroidism, immersion. Normally rewarm at a rate *not greater* than 1°C/h. Place on bed with electrically heated warming blanket. Wrap in a space-blanket. Place in a warm room (30±2°C). Stimulation must be kept to the minimum.

Monitor
1   Core temperature
2   Skin temperature
3   ECG
4   BG (corrected according to core temperature)
5   BG electrolytes
6   Right atrial pressure (RAP)
7   Urine output

Rewarm more actively under the following circumstances:
Acute immersion incident <30 min ago with core temperature <30°C
Core temperature <28°C
Core temperature continues to fall after 30 min of the above measures

In the acute immersion incident <30 min previously place the patient in a hot bath (temperature 42-45°C) without additional supportive therapy. Active rewarming is rarely instituted in an ITU.

Additional measures for rewarming include warming all intra-venous and gastric fluids to body temperature, heating inhalational gases to 41°C and humidifying to 100%.
More rapid rewarming may be obtained by peritoneal dialysis with fluids warmed to 38°C.

4.0 Specific problems

4.1 Disorders in body temperature

Treatment of complications
Hypoxia—oxygen via a face mask should be routine. IPPV (intermittent positive pressure ventilation) may occasionally be needed if PaO_2 falls to <6.0 kPa (45 mmHg).

Dehydration—polyuria is common—fluids should be titrated intravenously according to RAP. Plasma protein fraction (PPF) is the solution of choice since increased capillary permeability is a known complication.

Hypotension—generally due to displacement of central blood volume during rewarming—titrate fluids according to RAP.

Acidosis—maintain the correct pH at 7.3-7.4—this may necessitate aliquots of intravenous sodium bicarbonate (50 mmol). Observe for hypernatraemia.

Hyperglycaemia—actrapid insulin 4-8 units intravenously hourly if BG >10.0 mmol/l.

Arrhythmias—do not be concerned if there is a severe bradycardia or atrial fibrillation (AF). Ventricular fibrillation (VF) may be precipitated by stimulation and may revert spontaneously or with ECM (external cardiac massage). Anti-arrhythmic drugs are of little value. Perform ECM and rewarm with hot intravenous fluids and if necessary by exchange transfusion until core temperature is 28°C or greater. Generally spontaneously cardiovert, if not d.c. shock at low voltage (20-150 joules).

Shivering can be suppressed by heating the skin with a hot water blanket or if the patient is being ventilated by muscle relaxation.

Hyperthermia

Heat stroke
Most likely to occur in the presence of high ambient temperatures and increased relative humidity. Two groups of individuals most commonly affected are the debilitated and those with exertional heat stroke, usually the young. Exertional heat stroke is likely to occur when exercise is continued, when clothing is excessive, and when there is fatigue, pre-existent dehydration or obesity. Heat stroke may be drug-induced, the major mechanism for this being depression of the hypothalamic centres (Table 4.1).

4.0 Specific problems

4.1 Disorders in body temperatures

Clinical feature

There is a multisystem involvement depending upon the degree of destruction produced by the primary hyperthermia, tissue hypoxia secondary to haemodynamic failure and subsequent metabolic derangements.

Neurological	Disorientation → coma
	Ataxia
	Dysarthria
Haematological	DIC and increased fibrinolysis
	Microangiopathic haemolytic anaemia
Cardiac	Subendocardial haemorrhage may lead to infarction
	Cardiac enzymes increased
Hepatic	Centrilobular necrosis → jaundice
	Cholestasis → cholangitis
Renal	Acute intrinsic renal failure may develop in up to 25% of individuals with exertional heat stroke
	Myoglobinuria may occur
Musculo-skeletal	Exertional heat stroke potassium ↓ may go on to potassium ↑ due to muscle necrosis
Sweat glands	Sweating is often absent
Pulmonary	Lung haemorrhages and infarction are common

Treatment

This is described in Table 4.2.

Malignant hyperpyrexia

A rare condition developing during anaesthesia which occurs in individuals with an underlying disease of muscle. Since the condition occurs during anaesthesia instantaneous recognition by the anaesthetist is essential in order to save life. All anaesthetic agents are stopped immediately. Mycoplasmic calcium is reduced by i.v. dantrolene or, if not available, procaine hydrochloride 0.5 g/kg BW/min.

Active cooling should be instituted immediately. Hyperkalaemia is treated with dextrose insulin. A pH of <7.2 is an indication for the use of sodium bicarbonate 50 mmol aliquots every 15 min until the pH is >7.2. Excess sodium bicarbonate should be avoided. Further details of various aspects of malignant hyperpyrexia are available in the review article by Gronert (1980).

4.2 Management of acute metabolic disorders

Metabolic response to stress

Following acute stress there is an initial phase (ebb phase) where metabolism is reduced; this generally lasts several hours and is followed by a period of increased heat production and catabolism (flow phase). During the flow phase the following changes take place:

1 Transient elevation of body temperature.
2 Increased blood levels and increased urinary excretion of corticosteroids and catecholamines.
3 Increased blood levels of aldosterone and ADH (antidiuretic hormone).
4 Initial fall in insulin level followed by an elevation; the effect however is antagonized by catecholamines and corticosteroids with a tendency towards hyperglycaemia.
5 Increased levels of T_3 and T_4.
6 These metabolic changes are manifested as:
   - a catabolic phase with a negative nitrogen and caloric balance and loss of body weight (10% of the BW may be lost within 14 days), mobilization of free fatty acids and gluconeogenesis
   - oliguria with a tendency towards water retention
   - increased retention of sodium ions and a tendency towards an intracellular sodium shift
   - increased urinary loss of potassium, phosphate, calcium, magnesium and zinc
   - hyperglycaemia

These factors must be taken into account during the metabolic management of the stressed patient.

Management of acute disorders in water and sodium balance

The term dehydration is commonly used to denote sodium and water depletion when it should be confined to pure water depletion. The differentiation between dominant water and sodium depletion is of importance to ensure appropriate treatment (Table 4.3).

4.0 Specific problems

4.2 Management of acute metabolic disorders

Water depletion
Average water requirement is 20-40 ml/kg BW daily and depletion
may be related to decreased intake or increased losses (diarrhoea,
sweating, hyperventilation). Relative water depletion may occur
when normal saline has been used to replace hypotonic losses.

Management of water depletion
This is summarized in Table 4.4

Abnormalities in serum sodium concentration
True salt depletion and water intoxication are rare causes for a fall
in serum sodium (Table 4.5). The extracellular fluid is predominantly sodium-containing whereas the intracellular fluid
containts potassium ions. The ratio of sodium ions in the extracellular to the intracellular compartments is approximately 50:1;
the relationship can be markedly affected by stress and extreme
illness where sodium tends to shift into the cells. There is a close
relationship between serum sodium and osmolality. Diagnosis and
treatment of hyponatraemic states are summarized in Table 4.6.

Loss of total body sodium. The causes of losses of total body
sodium are enumarated in Table 4.5. When in doubt secretions
should be analysed—upper intestinal secretions have a sodium
content of around 80-150 mmol per litre (Table 4.7). The signs
and symptoms are described in the table on p. 174. Slight to
moderate sodium depletion represents a total body sodium deficit
of 8 mmol/kg and moderate to severe 8-11.5 mmol/kg BW.
Treatment is summarized in Table 4.8.

Dilutional hyponatraemia. The causes for dilutional hyponatraemia are described in Table 4.5, and treatment summarized
in Table 4.6.

Water intoxication
The condition is unlikely to develop in patients drinking spontaneously since nausea and distaste for water occurs early.
Patients under stress are particularly predisposed to the condition
because of high circulating levels of ADH. Patients with head
injury and pregnant patients with complications towards term and
at delivery are particularly predisposed to the condition. The
serum sodium is generally <120 mmol/l and the serum osmolality
decreased, the urinary sodium is variable. In the condition of
IADH (inappropriate release of antidiuretic hormone) syndrome
the serum sodium and osmolality are low and the urinary sodium
in the presence of oliguria >30 mmol/l.

144

4.0 Specific problems

4.2 Management of acute metabolic disorders

Treatment for water intoxication is summarized in Table 4.10.

Look for any factor producing *IADH syndrome* and treat appropriately.

Sodium shift: the sick cell syndrome
In the critically ill a falling serum sodium does not necessarily indicate a depletion of total body sodium and sodium ions must not be infused unless the diagnosis is certain.

Sodium shift is a bad prognostic sign, the serum sodium rising as the patient's condition improves. The rules are:
- only give sufficient sodium to replace that lost in urine, etc.
- restore circulating volume, correct hypotension and hypoxia
- do not overhydrate
- observe for renal failure and treat accordingly
- ensure that the patient is not potassium depleted
- consider the dextrose/insulin regime

Hypernatraemia
Aetiology, diagnosis and management, see the hyperosmolar states on p. 155.

Acute disorders in potassium balance

Potassium is the predominant cation of cells, its distribution being related to cell mass (approximately 83% being allocated in the muscle cell). A calculated negative balance of K ions does not necessarily mean a deficiency, this depending upon the capacity of the cells for potassium (increased when the protein and glycogen content of the cells is increased).

Kidneys' ability to conserve potassium (in contrast to sodium) is limited. Symptoms are more pronounced in acute potassium deficiency, there being less time to adjust the intracellular/extracellular potassium ratio. It is essential to relate the serum potassium to intracellular-extracellular shifts and factors affecting potassium shifts are summarized in Table 4.11. Factors producing a fall in total body potassium are enumerated in Table 4.12.

A 70 kg male on average has a total body potassium of 3800 mmol. Chronic potassium depletion is associated (in the presence of normal renal function) with urinary potassium of <10 mmol/l. With progressive K depletion renal conservation of K is often lost (this generally occurs after 3 weeks of K depletion). A metabolic alkalosis is suggestive of a non-renal cause for the hypokalaemia.

At least 10% of the total body K has to be lost before symptoms occur. These are frequently vague and include weakness, lassitude, thirst, anorexia progressing when severe to tetany, paresis and terminating in VF.

ECG changes are helpful in making the initial diagnosis but the rate of improvement may not correlate with the serum potassium.

Initially the S-T segment becomes depressed, the U wave exaggerated and the T wave amplitude decreased without changing the duration of the Q-T interval. The P and QRS amplitude and duration may be increased and the P-R interval prolonged (Fig. 4.1).

The combination of digoxin and quinidine may mimic the ECG changes of hypokalaemia. S-T segment depression generally is evident at serum potassium levels of 3.0-3.2 mmol/l with frank ECG changes at Se K of 2.8 mmol/l or less. At a serum concentration of K of 3.2 mmol/l or less ventricular and supraventricular ectopics are common and junctional or atrial tachycardia may develop at levels of 2.8-3.2 mmol/l with or without digoxin therapy. VF is likely to occur at levels of 2.5 mmol/l or less.

Treatment of hypokalaemia is summarized in Table 4.13.

Management of potassium excess
The causes for potassium excess are listed in Table 4.14.

The rate of rise in Se K in a catabolic patient with renal failure may be extremely rapid, the patient developing dangerous hyperkalaemia within 24 h of onset of renal failure.

K 2.8 mmol/l

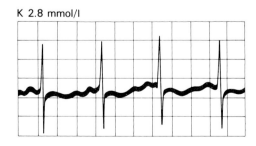

Fig. 4.1. ECG showing changes secondary to hypokalaemia.

4.0 Specific problems

4.2 Management of acute metabolic disorders

Succinylcholine may produce a lethal efflux of potassium from muscle in patients who have sustained thermal trauma, direct muscle trauma or are suffering from a neurological muscle deficit.

The neuromuscular effects rarely appear until the Se K is >8 mmol/l and include paraesthesiae, tingling around the mouth, hands and feet, burning and a numbness of the extremities and variable muscle paresis. Fixed dilated pupils have been reported.

A serum concentration of 8.5 mmol/l or more may be complicated by VF and cardiac arrest.

ECG changes in hyperkalaemia generally closely correlate with the Se K level (Fig. 4.2). The T wave peaks when the plasma K reaches 5.5 mmol/l, the QRS widens when the K exceeds 6.5 mmol/l, PR becomes prolonged at levels above 7.0 mmol/l. The T wave *may not peak* in hyperkalaemia.

K 7.0 mmol/l

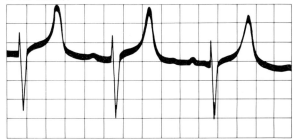

K 8.3 mmol/l

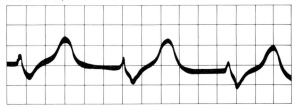

Fig. 4.2. ECG showing changes secondary to hyperkalaemia.

4.0 Specific problems

4.2 Management of acute metabolic disorders

Treatment
1 Identify the cause (Table 4.14).
2 Should the situation be readily reversible and renal function good, drug therapy may be sufficient (Table 4.15).
3 In renal failure, generally necessary to establish dialysis as soon as possible.
4 Best drug combination dextrose/insulin. Infuse 200 ml of 40% dextrose plus Actrapid insulin 16 units over 20-30 min. Check blood glucose before and 15 min after. Give Actrapid insulin 12 units i.v. if BG post infusion >12.0 mmol/l and monitor BG hourly repeating the insulin until BG <12.0 mmol/l.
5 When VF or serious dysrrhythmia has occurred calcium chloride should be given (Table 4.15). In renal failure, consider a continuous dextrose insulin infusion should the patient be haemodynamically unstable, since, under such circumstances dialysis is preferably delayed for 24 h. Avoid sodium bicarbonate should there be fluid overload or hypernatraemia.
6 The dextrose insulin regime may be used in patients in renal failure pre-operatively. During surgery the patient is hyperventilated and dialysis established postoperatively.
7 Exchange resin may be considered especially in patients on chronic dialysis where it has been decided to defer dialysis for 12-24 h. It is not suitable for catabolic patients.

Disorders of calcium and magnesium balance

The management of acute disorders of calcium metabolism is described in greater detail by Cohen (1978).

The body fluids contain only approximately 0.1% of the total body calcium. The level of serum calcium depends upon bowel absorption, renal excretion and bone excretion or resorption. 55-60% of the plasma calcium is ionized, most of the remainder being bound to protein.

The absorption of calcium is enhanced by Vitamin D.

Parathormone stimulates bone resorption and tubular resorption of calcium.

Hypocalcaemia
The causes of acute hypocalcaemia are summarized in Table 4.16

and are related to a lowered plasma ionized calcium, rare with total plasma calcium > 1.88 mmol/l.

Acute manifestations are tetany, carpopedal spasm and less frequently convulsions and laryngeal stridor.

Management of acute hypocalcaemia is summarized in Table 4.17.

Hypercalcaemia
The causes of hypercalcaemia are enumerated in Table 4.18.

Manifestations include polyuria, thirst, weakness, lassitude, anorexia, vomiting, constipation and mental confusion. When severe the presentation is that of a semicomatosed vomiting patient; a cardiac dysrhythmia is common and the level of serum calcium is generally > 3.75 mmol/l.

Treatment is summarized in Table 4.19.

Find the cause (Table 4.18), since in certain instances treating the underlying cause is the basis for treatment.

Evaluate renal function. Dialysis may be necessary if there is severely impaired renal function.

Avoid all calcium-containing solutions.

Insert a RAP line, restore volume with normal saline or PPF (increased renal clearance of sodium ions is associated with an increased clearance of calcium ions).

Correct a metabolic acidosis using sodium bicarbonate, 50 mmol bicarbonate ions in 100 ml of 1/5 normal saline infuse ½ hourly until pH > 7.3. *Do not use* sodium bocarbonate if Se K < 3.8 mmol/l. Avoid sodium and/or fluid overload. RAP restored to normal and urine output > 40 ml/h give 100 ml of 10% mannitol over 20 min, repeated 2 hourly until serum calcium < 2.8 mmol/l.

If hypokalaemia (K < 3.5 mmol/l) correct before using mannitol or sodium bicarbonate (Table 4.13).

Check serum magnesium, if low, correct (Table 4.21) monitor regularly, and once 0.70 mmol/l give 6-20 mmol daily as magnesium sulphate (Table 4.21).

4.0 Specific problems

4.2 Management of acute metabolic disorders

Specific therapy for hypercalcaemia is enumerated in Table 4.19.

Use frusemide where the patient will not tolerate fluid load alone or already has a high normal RAP at the onset of therapy. Careful monitoring of RAP and fluid balance is essential. Give 1 l of fluid every 3 h, generally ratio 4:1 1/5 normal saline to normal saline with potassium chloride 20 mmol/l.

Give frusemide 40-80 mg i.v. 4 hourly.

Monitor serum calcium, serum potassium 4-6 hourly.

Observe the ECG for hypokalaemia.

Stop infusion once serum calcium <2.7 mmol/l.

Serious cardiac dysrhythmia use i.v. dipotassium hydrogen phosphate. The infusion *must not be used* without ECG monitoring and resuscitation facilities. Too rapid infusion may precipitate calcium along the vein infused and/or a cardiac arrest. Commence infusion at 10 mmol phosphate (as dipotassium hydrogen phosphate 1 mmol phosphate/ml) in 100 ml 1/5 normal saline and infuse over 2 h. Slow down infusion rate if a bradyarrhythmia develops. Stop infusion once cardiac arrhythmia stops. Should a cardiac arrest have occurred intubate, hand ventilate, perform external cardiac massage and infuse 10 mmol of phosphate as above into a central line over 15 min.

Hypomagnesaemia
Only 1% of the total body magnesium is extracellular. The causes of *magnesium deficiency* are enumerated in Table 4.20. Magnesium deficiency is often associated with calcium and potassium depletion.

Clinical manifestations are vague and include weakness, tremors, coma, nausea and vomiting. Severe depletion (serum magnesium around 0.5 mmol/l) is associated with cardiac arrhythmias and tetany.

In the presence of an alkalosis (as with associated potassium depletion) tetany may occur at a higher level since the ionized fraction is decreased.

Treatment is summarized in Table 4.21.

4.0 Specific problems

4.2 Management of acute metabolic disorders

Phosphate depletion

Ratio of intracellular to extracellular phosphorus approximately
100:1. Serum phosphate may not reflect total bodystores.
Severe hypophosphataemia (serum phosphate <0.32 mmol/l)
may occur:
- during hyperalimentation
- nutritional recovery following starvation
- complicate renal dialysis
- chronic renal failure
- treatment of diabetic ketoacidosis

Manifestations of hypophosphataemia include muscle weakness,
hyperventilation (due to 2,3 DPG deficiency) haemolytic anaemia,
seizures and coma.

Treatment of severe hypophosphataemia is summarized in
Table 4.22. Phosphate infusions must be performed with careful
monitoring control when impaired renal function is present.

Acute disorders of acid base balance

The body attempts to maintain a pH between 7.38 and 7.42. pH
is an inverse and logarithmic expression of hydrogen ion concentration.

Hydrogen ion is present in the body in minute amount and is
heavily buffered. Its concentration is proportional to the ratio of
ventilatory function to metabolic function

$$[H_+] \propto \frac{PaCO_2}{[HCO_{3-}]}$$

Acid base disturbances are generally associated with other illnesses. The cause for the disturbance must be determined since
in many instances with correction of the basic cause the acid
base disturbance will correct spontaneously. It is important to
define the primary acid base abnormality since each acid base disturbance that occurs is associated with compensation; the second
parameter not responsible for the initial abnormality will also be
abnormal.

Respiratory acid base disorders are categorized in Table 4.23 and
metabolic disorders in Table 4.24.

4.0 Specific problems

4.2 Management of acute metabolic disorders

Metabolic acid base disturbances
Primary metabolic acidosis: The diagnosis can be assisted by
determining whether an anion gap is present.

$$[Na^+] - [(HCO_3^-) + (Cl^-)] = 5\text{-}12 \text{ mEq/l}$$

Normally the sum of residual anions (sulphates, phosphates, poly-
ionic plasma proteins and anions of organic acids) range from
5-12 mEq/l (Fig. 4.3a). In conditions of acidosis with a normal
anion gap there is a reduction of bicarbonate and compensatory
hyperchloraemia (Fig. 4.3b). In anion gap acidosis the bicarbonate
deficit is made up of an increased concentration of residual anions
(Fig. 4.3c).
Consequences of a metabolic acidosis are enumerated in
Table 4.25. The causes of a primary metabolic acidosis are
summarized in Table 4.26.

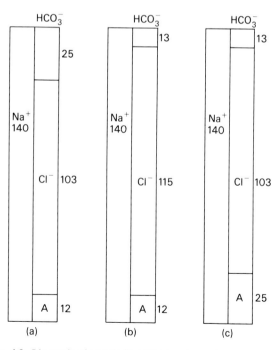

Fig. 4.3. Diagnosis of metabolic acidosis using anion gap.
(a) Normal pH; (b) pH normal anion gap; (c) pH increased anion
gap. A = residual anions.

4.0 Specific problems

4.2 Management of acute metabolic disorders

Treatment (other than lactic acidosis) is summarized in Table 4.27.

Lactic acidosis: Lactic acid is eliminated when the lactate ions are converted by the liver or kidney to glucose or oxidized. Either overproduction of failure of removal can result in lactic acidosis. Two types have been defined, type A and type B, and may be classified according to Table 4.28. Conditions which predispose the patient to lactic acidosis are shown in Table 4.29.
Type A is the type most commonly seen in the critically ill and occurs when there is evidence of tissue hypoxia. Treatment is summarized in Table 4.30.

Primary metabolic alkolosis: The disorders causing a metabolic alkalosis can be defined according to their response to sodium chloride administration. The factors, mechanisms and treatment of primary metabolic alkolosis likely to be seen in the critically ill are summarized in Table 4.31. A metabolic alkalosis (pH >7.5 and/or base excess >8.0) is potentially dangerous in any critically ill patient, the reasons being:

1 Often associated with total body potassium depletion
2 When associated with potassium depletion renal failure (impaired creatinine clearance and renal concentrating capacity) is common, increasing the susceptibility towards acute renal failure
3 May lead to compensatory respiratory depression particularly dangerous in any patient with respiratory failure
4 Adverse shift of the oxyhaemoglobin dissociation curve requiring an increase in cardiac output in order to maintain adequate oxygen delivery to the peripheral cell.

Treatment is summarized in Table 4.31.
Gastric aspirate can generally be replaced volume for volume by normal saline plus appropriate potassium replacement. Large volumes of aspirate should be analysed for sodium content. Pyloric obstruction should be treated by gastric drainage, insertion of a RAP line and infusion of normal saline and potassium chloride until the RAP is up to 4 cm of water. This may require many litres of normal saline. No operation should be contemplated until the metabolic deficits have been corrected.
Consider the use of arginine monohydrochloride when a metabolic alkalosis develops following the overuse of bicarbonate under the following circumstances:

- pH >7.55 (base excess >10) in the presence of respiratory depression and pulmonary pathology in a patient breathing spontaneously
- pH >7.5 (base excess >10) in the presence of hypoxia in particular when there is limited cardiac reserve

The dose should be calculated according to the following formula correcting to a base excess of 10:

Number of H^+ required = kg BW $\times 0.3$ (base excess -10) as arginine monohydrochloride.

Arginine monohydrochloride $(C_6H_{14}N_4O_2HCl)$ 60% solution 140 mmol H^+/50 ml.

Use 1/5 normal saline as a carrier medium infusing at a rate of 30 mmol/h.

Disorders of uric acid metabolism

Hyperuricaemia may develop during the management of the critically ill under the following conditions:

- idiopathic gout
- myeloproliferative disease and reticulosis, in particular during cytotoxic therapy
- haemolytic states
- drugs — diuretics particularly in the gouty subject
- renal failure
- ketoacidosis associated with chronic starvation or diabetes mellitus

Acute uric acid obstruction of the urinary tract is the only problem likely to be encountered in the ITU.

Most patients treated by renal dialysis experience a diuresis within 48 h and once the serum urate is < 1.5 mmol/l. Dialysis should be started as soon as the diagnosis is made since delay may prolong the period of tubular obstruction.

Acute disorders of porphyrin metabolism

Characteristic of the porphyrias is the excess production of porphyrins or their precursors which can be measured in the faeces, blood or urine. The normal values and the porphyrias likely to be encountered in the critically ill are shown in Table 4.32.

The disease most likely to be seen is acute intermittent porphyria. Certain drugs or factors may precipitate or aggravate the condition (Table 4.33). The classic symptoms of an acute attack are abdominal and extremity pain, constipation and mental changes. BP swings, tachycardia, sweating, mental confusion, seizures and paresis of the bulbar and peripheral musculature may occur.

4.0 Specific problems

4.2 Management of acute metabolic disorders

Variations in BG and hyponatraemia are common.

Treatment is summarized in Table 4.34.

The hyperosmolar states

Normal serum osmolality 275-295 mosmol/kg. Calculated by the following equation:

$$Osmolality = 2Na \ (mmol/l) + glucose \ (mmol/l) + 2 \ BUN \ (mmol/l).$$

Biochemical estimation generally based on the fact that the unit mosmol/kg varies linearly with freezing point depression. In the critically ill the calculated level is often lower than the estimated level. The characteristics of disturbances of intracellular and extracellular volume and osmolality are shown in Table 4.35.

Factors which may cause an elevated osmolality include hyperglycaemia and hypernatraemia. Urea equilibrilates in all body spaces and therefore the hyperosmolar effects are not so dramatic as with glucose or sodium unless the rate of rise is rapid.

The stressed patient is particularly predisposed to the condition and the condition may be precipitated by various factors singly or in combination (Table 4.36).

Diminished urinary sodium excretion is particularly common in the critically ill, increasing the tendancy towards hypernatraemia.

Hyperosmolar syndromes unrelated to diabetes mellitus
In conscious patients an acute rise in serum osmolality produces a rapid onset of drowsiness followed by twitching, convulsions and ultimately respiratory arrest. In the acute syndrome, dehydration may not be present and there may be acute expansion of the intravascular space LV (left ventricular) overload and pulmonary oedema. Renal and respiratory failure is common. Serum osmolality >350 mosmol/kg is potentially fatal.

DIC may be a complication.

Management
1   Hyperosmolar syndrome of slow onset: serum osmolality
    <350 mosmol/kg.

4.0 Specific problems

4.2 Management of acute metabolic disorders

This does not require dramatic treatment and may be treated (depending upon whether the condition is predominantly hypernatraemia or hyperglycaemia) according to Table 4.37

2 Hyperosmolar syndrome of acute onset or serum osmolality >350 mosmol/kg in a hyperosmolar syndrome of chronic onset:

(a) Predominant hypernatraemia (see Table 4.38). When this is due to excessive infusion of Na^+ the serum sodium will reflect the gravity of the situation. With oral ingestion there may be a delayed rise in serum sodium and the rise estimated according to the following:

$$\text{Expected rise in Se } Na^+ \text{ (mmol/l)} = \frac{\text{total vol. of initial gastric aspirate (l)} \times \text{Na}^+ \text{ conc. in initial gastric aspirate (mmol/l)}}{\text{TBW (l) (Total body water)}}$$

(Table 4.39)

Should the expected rise be >20 mmol/l then peritoneal dialysis should be commenced.

(b) Predominant hyperglycaemia (unassociated with diabetes mellitus). A rapid rise in blood glucose can generally be adequately controlled with insulin therapy coupled with intravenous hypotonic or isotonic saline.

Treatment is summarized in Table 4.40

Hyperosmolar syndromes associated with diabetes mellitus
There is an overlap between the diabetic with non-ketotic hyperglycaemia (NKA) and the patient with classic diabetic ketoacidosis (Table 4.41).

1 Diabetic ketoacidosis (Table 4.42): The essential cause of diabetic ketoacidosis (DKA) is insufficiency of insulin leading to hyperglycaemia, raised levels of fatty acids in the blood and consequently ketoacidosis. The total electrolyte and water losses have been estimated as:

Water	75-100 ml/kg
Na^+	8 mmol/kg BW
Cl^-	5 mmol/kg BW
K^+	6 mmol/kg BW

A high serum sodium is evidence of extreme dehydration and is a precursor of imminent cardiovascular collapse from hypovolaemia.

4.0 Specific problems

4.2 Management of acute metabolic disorders

Treatment is summarized in Table 4.42.

Use PPF when hypotension is severe.

Do not give insulin or sodium bicarbonate if hypokalaemia is suspected. pH 7.1 or less is an indication for use of sodium bicarbonate.

Refractory acidosis, consider lactic acidosis; a sodium bicarbonate infusion may be necessary (Table 4.30).

Give insulin initially as an infusion or as i.v. boluses, changing to i.m. injections if preferred once perfusion improved.

Consider the use of heparin if refractory acidosis associated with clinical evidence of poor peripheral perfusion and haematological evidence of DIC.

RAP monitoring and sequestered biochemical monitoring essential.

2 Non-ketotic hyperglycaemia and diabetes mellitus (NKA):
Generally occurs in the elderly, may be an undiagnosed diabetic. Often a history of stress associated with a period of inadequate renal perfusion (e.g. congestive cardiac failure, hypoxia, hypovolaemia). May be precipitated by excessive ingestion of hypertonic solutions (e.g. alcohol, Lucozade). Degree of overlap with DKA common features shown in Table 4.41. BG generally >35 mmol/l and serum osmolality >340 mosm/kg.

Treatment summarized in Table 4.43.

Prognosis often poor because of age, organ failure, and level of osmolality with resultant permanent cerebral damage.

4.3 Management of endocrine crises

The thyroid gland

Both extreme underactivity and overactivity can lead to a medical emergency.

Myxoedema coma
This occurs in a patient with long-standing hypothyroidism generally >65 years. The precipitating factors and manifestations are enumerated in Tables 4.44 and 4.45 respectively.

Treatment is summarized in Table 4.46.

Treatment must be gradual—mortality is high, complications of treatment include myocardial infarction, cardiac failure, secondary infection.

Thyroid crisis (thyroid storm)
1 Mortality rate almost 100%.
2 Precipitating factors include surgery, administration of radio-active iodine in a patient inadequately prepared by pre-treatment with anti-thyroid drugs.
3 Manifestations are enumerated in Table 4.47.
4 The most important aspects of treatment are reduction of the hypercatabolic state and control of cardiac dysrhythmias.
5 Treatment is summarized in Table 4.48.

The adrenal gland

Addisonian crisis
Hypoadrenalism is of insidious onset, the crisis being precipitated by stress (trauma, surgery, infection). Hot weather, sweating and sodium loss are potent precipitating factors. Crisis may occur in patients on long-term steroids or on replacement therapy. Manifestations are listed in Table 4.49 and treatment summarized in Table 4.50.

Acute hypercortisolism
1 May arise in severe and long-term Cushing's syndrome and where there is ectopic adrenocorticol stimulating hormone (ACTH) production (e.g. bronchial carcinoma).
2 Manifestations are secondary to a hypokalaemic metabolic alkalosis which may be complicated by muscle weakness and cardiac dysrhythmias.

3 Plasma cortisol generally >2000 nmol/l.
4 ACTH low with primary adrenal gland lesions and high in ectopic ACTH production.
5 Treatment is summarized in Table 4.51.

Phaeochromocytoma
May be discovered in the routine investigations of hypertension but more commonly presents with sudden release of adrenaline noradrenaline. The presentation depends upon whether α-receptors (stimulated by adrenaline), or β-receptors (stimulated by noradrenaline) are affected (Table 4.52), often the presentation is mixed.

Suspect in any patient where tachycardia and peripheral vasoconstriction is extreme for no particular reason.

Precipitating factors include any form of stress
• general anaesthetic
• infection
• abdominal palpation
• contrast radiography

Patients may be extremely sensitive to β-blockade and may arrest as a result of their use.

Phaeochromocytoma commonly seen in relation to other disorders
• neurofibromata
• café au lait pigmentation
• meningiomata
• medullary carcinoma of the thyroid
• hyperparathyroidism
• diabetes mellitus
• carcinoid tumour
• multiple phaeochromocytoma

Diagnosis confirmed in an emergency by raised urinary catecholamines in acute severe hypertension; an intravenous phentolamine test is useful. Treatment is summarized in Table 4.53 and depends upon the receptors involved (Table 4.52).

Pituitary gland and hypothalamus

Hypopituitary coma
Generally insidious but may occur acutely in pituitary infarction or the chronic condition becomes acute because of stress.

Manifestations are summarized in Table 4.54.

Treatment is summarized in Table 4.55.

Disorders of ADH secretion
The ADH of man is arginine vasopressin (AVP) which is synthesized in the supraoptic and paraventricular nuclei.

Plasma osmolality is the main determinant of vasopressin release.

Diabetes insipidus (DI)
Polyuria results from
- deficiency of AVP (cranial diabetes insipidus (CDI)
- renal resistance to AVP (nephrogenic DI)
- excessive water intake

Causes are enumerated in Table 4.56.

Diagnosis is based on U/P osmolality ratio, water deprivation test and response to vasopressin (Bayliss 1981).

Treatment is summarized in Table 4.57.

4.4 Management of acute disorders of the nervous system (other than head injury)

Purulent meningitis

The cause is age-dependent except when the patient is immunologically depressed, when a wide variety of organisms may be involved.

The causes of meningitis are shown in Table 4.58.

In severe cases headache, nausea and neck stiffness may not be present—the patient may present with shock and circulatory collapse.

CSF is classically turbid
- WBC $>1000/\mu l>80\%$ polymorphonuclears
- protein >1000 mg/l
- glucose <2.1 mmol/l
- organisms may be present

Treatment is summarized in Table 4.59.

4.0 Specific problems

4.4 The nervous system

Status epilepticus

Any seizure type may carry on serially. All need urgent treatment—the patient may sustain permanent brain damage if status epilepticus is not corrected rapidly.

In a known epileptic, precipitating factor(s) should be eliminated and blood levels taken to check that the patient is taking the drug/s and that they are within the therapeutic range (Tables 4.60 and 4.61 respectively).

Treatment is summarized in Table 4.62.

Diazepam in high dosage is a respiratory depressant, ventilation must therefore be observed with care.

Where respiratory depression is of concern paraldehyde is a safer drug to use.

Acute polyneuropathies

The acute onset neuropathies include:
- Guillain-Barré syndrome
- porphyria
- diptheria
- toxic (in particular heavy metal and orthocresyl phosphate poisoning)
- post-vaccinial
- malignancy

The condition most commonly requiring treatment in the ITU is the Guillain-Barré syndrome but other causes must be excluded.

The Guillain-Barré syndrome may come on acutely with minimal peripheral neuropathy, progressing to respiratory paresis within hours. In others, progress is more insidious.

Diagnosis is made on the history and clinical findings. The CSF protein is generally elevated and cell concentration normal. In some patients protein may be normal and cells >30 cells/mm^3. CSF changes may not be present at the onset of the illness.

Treatment is summarized in Table 4.63.

Autonomic dysfunction is common in severe cases and requires skilled management.

Myasthenia gravis

A disease of unknown aetiology characterized by impairment of transmission at the motor neurone junctions in skeletal muscle. Two types of crisis may develop.

Myasthenic crisis
This may occur in the unknown myasthenic or in a myasthenic on inadequate treatment. It is precipitated by stress or infection.

Cholinergic crisis
This is caused by excess anticholinesterase medication in a known myasthenic.

Treatment of a myasthenic crisis
Diagnosis is confirmed by the edrophonium chloride (Tensilon) test. Edrophonium chloride 1-2 mg given i.v.; if no side-effects give 5-8 mg i.v. A positive response is indicated by an obvious improvement in strength within 1 min and lasting up to 5 min. Improvement in strength is shown by
- diminution in ptosis
- increase in time when the arm can be stretched
- improved vital capacity
Treatment is summarized in Table 4.64.

Treatment of a cholinergic crisis
This condition is caused by excess anticholinesterase medication and is confirmed by lack of response to edrophonium chloride.

Treatment is summarized in Table 4.65.

Brain stem death

This is a condition where the brain stem is no longer functioning and oxygenation (and hence cardiac activity) can only be maintained by artificial ventilation.

The condition must be differentiated from other causes of deep coma and having excluded these causes the criteria for brain stem death must all be present and verified by two senior doctors (one a consultant and the other a consultant or senior registrar) on two consecutive occasions.

The following factors are essential for diagnosis
1 The cause for the brain stem damage must be irremediable.
2 Coma must *not* be due to drugs (including muscle relaxants), hypothermia (core temperature >35°C), metabolic or endocrine disturbances.
3 Having excluded these causes the brain stem criteria are:
   - pupils both fixed to light
   - corneal reflexes absent
   - no eye movements on cold caloric testing
   - no cranial nerve motor responses
   - no gag reflexes
   - no respiratory movements on disconnecting the patient from the ventilator at a $PaCO_2$ of 6.7 kPa (50 mmHg) or above.
4 Recovery has never been known once brain stem death has occurred—the relatives should be consulted and the situation explained with a view to termination of artificial ventilation.
5 Further reading should include Posner (1978) Jennett (1981) Pallis (1982) and Working Party on behalf of the Health Departments of Great Britain and Northern Ireland (1983).

4.5 Management of gastro-intestinal emergencies

Massive gastro-intestinal haemorrhage

The severity of haemorrhage can be assessed according to the clinical signs (p. 115) and volume replacement is based on the advice given on p. 95.

Patients with an episode of severe haemorrhage should be admitted to the ITU and management conducted according to Table 4.66.

Inflammatory bowel disease

A patient may be admitted to the ITU with severe acute diarrhoea —early diagnosis is imperative in order to establish correct treatment (Table 4.67).

Acute ulcerative colitis
A patient may be admitted in his/her first acute attack or may sustain an acute relapse.

Diagnosis should be confirmed by sigmoidoscopy.

Management is summarized in Table 4.68.

Acute severe Crohn's disease
May be difficult to diagnose. May present with fever, diarrhoea, rectal bleeding, abdominal pain or even perforation.

Diagnosis may be confirmed in 30% of patients by emergency histology of rectal biopsy material.

Radiology of small and large bowel may be necessary.

Treatment is summarized in Table 4.69.

Acute severe pancreatitis

Mortality rate for acute pancreatitis requiring intensive therapy is as high as 80%.

Pancreatitis may not be diagnosed until after laparotomy (the amylase level is *not always* raised).

Indications for admission to an ITU are enumerated in Table 4.70.

Acute early complications of pancreatitis are enumerated in Table 4.71.

Pulmonary failure is common and is associated with a poor prognosis: early ventilation is recommended.

Treatment is summarized in Table 4.72 and specific aspects of management in Table 4.73.

Patients with severe acute pancreatitis may take many months to recover and weeks may be spent in the ITU, the patient requiring supportive care.

4.6   Treatment of poisoning

Introduction

The majority of intoxications are admitted to the wards; patients requiring intensive therapy maybe suffering from the following:

4.0 Specific problems

4.6 Poisoning

- loss of airway control
- organ failure
- an intoxication which may have dangerous late effects (e.g. cardiac dysrrhythmia)

General treatment (Table 4.74)

Certain basic therapeutic principles apply to the majority of poisons.

Airway control is esstential.

Where hypoventilation is suspected an Astrup analysis is essential, since hypoxia and a respiratory acidosis may increase the incidence of cardiac dysrrhythmias. The PaO_2 in a patient with no previous history of respiratory disease should be maintained above 9.3 kPa (70 mmHg). Where aspiration is suspected, the patient should be electively intubated and ventilated using a muscle relaxant if necessary.

A degree of hypotension (80-100 mmHg SP) often does not require specific therapy. A RAP should be inserted and where myocardial depression is likely maintained at 2-4 cm H_2O.

Do not use inotropes unless urine output and/or peripheral perfusion are poor. Isoprenaline in general should be avoided unless its β-adrenergic effect is required (e.g. β-blocker overdose).

Dobutamine is the inotrope of choice. Use dopamine if urine output is poor.

Cardiac tachyarrhythmias should *not be* treated unless there is imminent danger of VF or tachycardia or the dysrrhythmia has produced a serious fall in cardiac output (CO). Dysrrhythmias related to tricylics should be treated with sodium bicarbonate (25-50 mmol i.v. over 5 min as required). Respiratory acidosis should be avoided — by ventilation if necessary.

Use antidysrrhythmics with *extreme care*, especially β-blockers, but most may precipitate an asystolic arrest. d.c. cardioversion is a preferable manoeuvre for ventricular tachycardia, lignocaine titrated slowly i.v. is probably the safest antidysrrhythmic (p. 71).

4.0 Specific problems

4.6 Poisoning

Bradycardia is an indication for insertion of a temporary pacemaker if:

- pulse rate <70/min and ECG evidence of heart block
- pulse rate <60/min and multiple ventricular ectopic beats are present
- pulse rate <50/min when a myocardial depressant or digoxin has been ingested and/or the haemodynamic state is likely to deteriorate

Hypothermia is common; generally reward slowly (p. 140).

Gastric lavage should be performed in all patients where ingestion has been <4 h and up to 12 h in patients who have ingested atropine type compounds, antidepressants, salicylates and digoxin. Where the airway is in doubt perform with an endotracheal tube in position.

Adsorbents may be considered for certain drugs. They are administered after gastric washout and are put down the Ryles tube. Refined activated charcoal (Medicoal) is generally used. Aspiration of these compounds may be dangerous.

Mantain the acid base and metabolic balance as near normal as possible. Do not start a forced alkaline diuresis until the Se K is >3.6 mmol/l. Ensure that the pH and $PaCO_2$ are kept normal in patients with tricyclic overdose.

Check the metabolic effects of specific drugs and correct as quickly as possible (e.g. diuretics, salicylates). Observe urine output and renal function if hypotension is prolonged or the drug ingested is potentially nephrotoxic.

Spasm in tricyclic overdose may impair ventilation; intubation and ventilation using a muscle relaxant should be considered. Epanutin is the drug of choice for convulsions but if severe and uncontrollable, low dose diazepam should be used. The use of diazepam may necessitate ventilation because of the respiratory depressant effect.

Antidotes—these are few. Naloxone hydrochloride (up to 0.4 mg titrated slowly intravenously until respiratory depression reversed) is effective against opioids. The effect is temporary and may have to be repeated. In large narcotic overdose it is far safer to intubate and ventilate. Cobalt edetate (20 ml of 1.5% solution in glucose) will counteract cyanide intoxication if given soon enough. Methionine or cysteine may be used for paracetamol overdose (see below). Desferrioxamine mesylate should be used in acute iron intoxication. Organ failure support is discussed elsewhere.

Certain aspects, however, should be mentioned:

1. Renal failure is non-catabolic and can often be treated conservatively unless drug clearance is dependent upon renal function.
2. Liver failure in paracetamol overdose may present with hypoglycaemia. Blood glucose monitoring and dextrose infusions are therefore important.
3. DIC and coagulation failure may occur when hypotension and hypoperfusion has been prolonged—clotting factor replacement is generally all that is necessary.
4. Haemodialysis is rarely indicated except in renal failure where peritoneal dialysis is not possible.
5. Haemoperfusion has had its advocates and is still under investigation.

The majority of poisonings are treated along traditional lines.

Particular aspects of management of the more common poisonings

Forced alkaline diuresis
Consider its use in severe intoxication due to the poisons enumerated in Table 4.75.

Dangers are:
- fluid overload
- hypokalaemia, hyperkalaemia
- metabolic alkalosis

Dangers eliminated by the use of a RAP line and careful monitoring.

Method summarized in Table 4.76.

Forced acid diuresis
This is rarely used but consider its use in severe intoxication due to chlorpromazine. The method is described by Stone & Wright (1978).

4.0 Specific problems

4.6 Poisoning

Specific management

Poisoning with β-blockers
1 Gastric lavage up to 10 h after ingestion.
2 Insert a RAP line if > 10 cmH₂O and hypotension present. Consider insertion of a PCWP probe.
3 RAP high PCWP high and BP↓ with oliguria commence an isoprenaline infusion. Titrate intravenously (5-30 μg/min) untill BP SP 80 mm or higher — the dosage required may be high. Failure to respond, use adrenaline or dobutamine.
4 Bradycardia in the absence of hypotension give i.v. atropine. Should it fail to raise pulse rate > 50/min insert a pacemaker.
5 Bronchospasm will respond to steroids and aminophylline (when serious haemodynamic manifestations are absent) or isoprenaline.
6 Observe fluid balance, keep fluids to < 1500 ml daily. Left heart failure is a common complication.
7 Consider ventilation if LVF or hypoxia is present. Ventilation may seriously reduce CO. PCWP and CO monitoring is advisable.

Poisoning with tricyclic antidepressants
1 Gastric washout up to 24 h after ingestion.
2 ECG monitor and continue until QRS complex < 100 msec for > 12 h.
3 Rising $PaCO_2$ and pH < 7.35 intubate and ventilate. Maintain $PaCO_2$ around 3.0 kPa. Maintain pH 7.35-7.45.
4 Arrhythmias *do not* treat unless CO, compromised generally, resolve with sodium bicarbonate 25-50 mmol i.v. On rare occasions small bolus doses of lignocaine may be necessary.
5 Convulsions and severe tremors — intubate with a muscle relaxant and ventilate, consider low dose diazepam.

Paracetamol overdose
The admission plasma-paracetamol level estimated as an emergency and related to the time of ingestion is used as a guide to the need for treatment (Fig. 4.4).

The antidote should be given within 12 h of ingestion. This consists of methionine (2.5 g via Ryles tube followed by three further doses 4 hourly) or cysteine (150 mg/kg by slow i.v. infusion then 50 mg/kg i.v. over 4 h followed by 100 mg/kg i.v. over 6 h).

The signs of liver failure generally develop 2-3 days later and

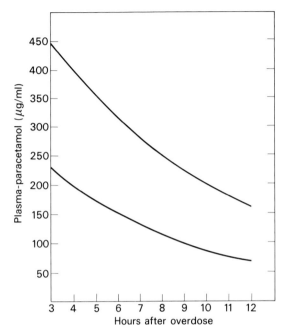

Fig. 4.4. Plasma-paracetamol concentrations in relationship to time after overdose. Liver damage is likely to be severe above the upper line, severe to mild between the lines, and clinically insignificant under the line. Treat with methionine or cysteine above the lower line (from Prescott et al. 1976).

should be treated as described on pp. 55-59. Hypoglycaemia may develop within 24 h of ingestion.

Salicylate intoxication
The complications are multiple and largely metabolic and respiratory. Other rarer complications include gastric ulceration or perforation, a haemorrhagic diathesis, cardiac dysrrhythmias, cardiac failure and renal failure. Sequential biochemical and haematological monitoring is essential.

Management is summarized in Table 4.77.

Acute digitalis poisoning
1 Peak serum digoxin level of >25 ng/ml >6 h after ingestion

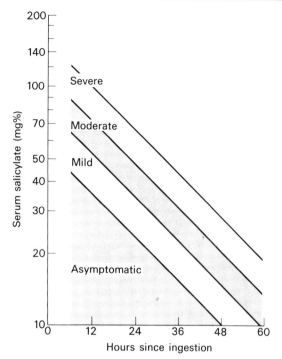

Fig. 4.5. Normogram relating serum salicylate concentration and expected severity of intoxication at varying intervals following ingestion of a single dose of salicylate (after Done, 1960).

   is likely to be fatal (fatalities may occur at lower levels).
2 Admission Se K >5.5 mmol/l is generally fatal.
3 Management is summarized in Table 4.78.
4 ECG monitoring is essential. Progress may be assessed by serial plasma digoxin levels.

Organophosphorus poisoning
These compounds are powerful anticholinesterase agents, the clinical effects being of cholinergic excess. Death is from respiratory failure due to laryngospasm, bronchoconstriction complicated by increased tracheobronchial and salivary secretions. Diagnosis is confirmed by blood cholinesterase estimation.

Treatment is summarized in Table 4.79.

4.0 Specific problems

4.6 Poisoning

Total recovery may take several months.

Paraquat poisoning
This is a dipyridylium weedkiller or herbicide — cutaneous exposure or inhalation rarely causes poisoning, swallowing 10-15 ml of the liquid concentrate or two to three satchets of the granules may be fatal.

Trade names likely to be encountered in the UK are:
- Dextrone*
- Dexuron*
- Esgram*
- Gramonol*
- Gramoxone*
- Gramoxone S*
- Pathclear
- Terraklene*
- Tota-Col*
- Weedol

* Most fatalities caused by these concentrated preparations.

Suspect in any patient with ulceration of the mouth presenting with multi-system failure which is followed by progressive pulmonary failure.

Outcome can be related to the time after ingestion (Fig. 4.6). Patients above the line are unlikely to survive.

Management is summarized in Table 4.80.

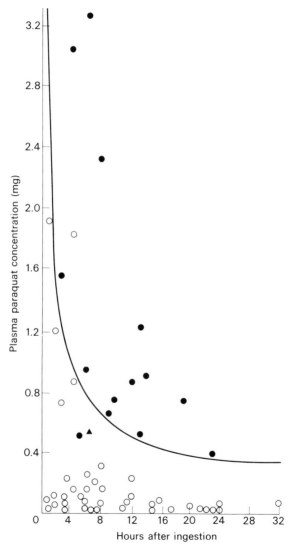

Fig. 4.6. Plasma paraquat concentrations in forty-four patients related to time after ingestion and outcome. ●, *Death;* ○, *survival;* ▲, *aspiration death.*
(From Proudfoot *et al.*, 1979)

Table 4.1. Drugs which may predispose to heat stroke

Phenothiazines
Antihistamines
Tricyclic antidepressants
Belladonna alkaloids
Glutethimide
Alcohol
Amphetamine abuse
Chronic diuretic therapy leading to dehydration

Table 4.2. Treatment of heat stroke

1 Remove all clothing
2 Pack body with ice and massage the skin to encourage heat dissipation
3 Cool body with fans
4 Shivering—suppress with intramuscular chlorpromazine
5 Lavage the stomach with iced water
6 Intubate and ventilate under the following circumstances:
   • loss of airway control
   • deep coma and danger of aspiration
   • uncontrollable shivering
   • convulsions
   • extensive lung pathology
   • $PaCO_2$ <9.0 kPa (67.5 mmHg)
7 Fluid volume replacement should be with PPF according to the RAP. A low blood pressure in the presence of a normal RAP may be an indication for insertion of a pulmonary capillary wedge pressure catheter
8 Low CO in the presence of normovalaemia may be an indication for an inotrope (p. 77). Electrolyte balance— dextrose insulin may be required if serum potassium >6.0 mmol/l
9 DIC—replace clotting factors with FFP, consider low dose heparin (p. 129)
10 Acute renal failure—rising serum potassium may be an indication for peritoneal dialysis. The body temperature may be further lowered by using cold dialysate

4.7 Tables

11 Convulsions—use phenytoin sodium, sedate and ventilate if uncontrollable.
12 *Stop cooling* once the temperature is 38.5°C since the patient may become hypothermic.

Table 4.3. Comparison between pure water and sodium depletion

Symptoms	Pure water depletion	Pure sodium depletion
Thirst	Present	Absent
Headache	Absent	Present
Lassitude	Mild, develops late	Early, progressive, severe
Muscle cramps	Absent	Present
Signs		
Temperature	High	Normal
Skin	Dry flushed, normal elasticity, doughy	Inelastic, loose and wrinkled
Blood pressure	Normal until late	Low
Biochemistry		
Urine volume	Diminished	Normal until late
osmolality	Increased	Decreased
chloride	Normal	Low except in Addison's disease
Blood PCV	Normal until late	Decreased
osmolality	Normal or increased	Decreased
sodium	Increased	Normal or decreased
urea	Slight increase	Moderate or severe increase

Table 4.4. Management of water depletion

Moderate deficit
1 Replace fluid with 5% dextrose or, where there have been minor sodium losses, 1/5 normal saline.

Severe depletion (where BP is falling)
1 Insert RAP line
2 Infuse 1/5 normal saline approximately 1 litre hourly until RAP >2 cm H_2O and BP >100 mm SP. Slow down infusion rate once this has been achieved so that the total estimated loss is replaced over the subsequent 24 h plus the continuing losses.

continued

Table 4.4—*continued*

3 Observe urine output (oliguria common, avoid overload). ARF rare
4 Observe for a fall in serum potassium and replace as necessary
5 *Do not* use dextrose 5% if Se K <3.3 mmol/l
6 Check Ca^{2+} Mg^{2+} may require replacement in patients with gastro-intestinal losses or prolonged glycosuria
7 Observe acid base state—an increasing metabolic alkalosis often indicates a fall in total body potassium

Table 4.5. Causes of a low serum sodium

Loss of total body sodium

Renal	Osmotic diuretics
	Diuretic therapy
	Renal disease
	Adrenal insufficiency
Gastro-intestinal	Vomiting
	Intestinal fluid loss
	Intestinal stasis
Skin	Excessive sweating (rare in temperate climate)
	Burns
Drainage	Pleural
	Peritoneal
	Other

Dilutional (normal total body sodium)

Water intoxication	Use of syntocinon
	Use of high volumes of hypotonic solution in the presence of oliguria
Colonic or bladder washouts with water	Post-stress states
	Inappropriate secretion of ADH
Fluid shift	Mannitol
	Glucose

Sodium shift (normal or increased total body sodium)
Hypokalaemia
Sick cell syndrome

Table 4.6. Diagnosis and treatment of hyponatraemic states

Diagnosis	Extra-renal sodium loss	Renal sodium loss	Dilutional states	Sodium shift
History and aetiology	Evidence of excessive non-renal sodium loss	Evidence of renal disease, or Addison's disease	1 Evidence of decreased renal water clearance Excessive hypotonic fluid administration in the presence of oliguria 2 IADH 3 Fluid shift, e.g. mannitol glucose	Oedematous states Hypokalaemia Patient suffering from a critical illness e.g. sepsis, trauma, cardiogenic, septic or hypovolaemic shock.
ECF volume	Decreased	Decreased	Increased	Normal or increased
Urine sodium conc.	<30 mmol/l	>30 mmol/l	1 generally >30 mmol/l 2 >30 mmol/l	<30 mmol/l

continued

Table 4.6—*continued*

Treatment		
Saline replacement therapy Corticosteroid for Addison's disease	1 Treatment of renal failure Restriction of fluid administration	Oedematous states Consider diuretics Sodium and water restriction
	2 IADH syndrome—consider corticosteroids Treatment of factors producing IADH syndrome	Hypokalaemia Potassium replacement Sick cell syndrome Treat the cause Sodium replacement not indicated
	3 Fluid shift Mannitol, consider dialysis if fluid overload and no diuresis Glucose give insulin	

Table 4.7. Average range of electrolyte concentration (mmol/l) of intestinal fluids in normal adults and the approximate maximum relative loss per 24 h

	Na^+	K^+	Cl^-	Approximate maximum fluid loss per 24 h (l)
Stomach	20-116	5-32	50-154	20
Bile	130-160	3-12	80-120	1.5
Pancreatic juice	110-150	3-10	54-95	1.5
Small bowel (suction)	72-148	2-15	43-137	6.0
Ileostomy (recent)	105-144	6-29	90-136	3.0
Cecostomy	45-115	11-28	35-70	3.0
Formed stool	10	10	15	0.2
Watery diarrhoea	50-100	20-40	40-80	17.0

4.0 Specific problems

Table 4.8. Treatment of depletion of total body sodium

1 Establish that the patient has true depletion in total body sodium
2 Analyse secretions and urine for sodium content
3 Assess total sodium loss by history, fluid balance charts and secretion analysis
4 A guide to the quantity of sodium ions lost can be estimated (see following table)

Rate of sodium replacement
1 Severe depletion (hypotension RAP <0 cmH$_2$O oliguria) give twice normal saline at a rate not >2 mmol Na$^+$ m^2 body surface/min until RAP 1.0 cmH$_2$O and to a maximum total of 300 mmol
   See table below for body surface area*
2 Then continue with normal saline infusing to a RAP of 2-4 cmH$_2$O and a BP SP >100 mm of mercury

Moderate to severe depletion
1 Use normal saline infusing until the RAP 2-4 cmH$_2$O and a BP SP >100 mmHg.
2 In moderate or severe sodium depletion where a low serum albumin (<30 g/l) is likely at least 50% of the replacement should be as PPF
3 Check acid base periodically, since in the presence of renal failure some of the sodium replacement should be given as sodium bicarbonate
4 In the presence of moderate sodium depletion and where renal volume handling is poor, 100-200 mmol of sodium ions may be given as twice normal saline or as 8.4% sodium bicarbonate.

Weight (kg)	Surface area (m^2)
30	1.05
40	1.30
50	1.50
60	1.65
70	1.75
80	1.85
90	1.95
100	2.05

*Simplified table for body surface area

4.0 Specific problems

4.7 Tables

Attempt to replace ⅓ to ½ of the estimated loss plus current losses over the first 12 h replacing totally within 24 h.

5 Observe serum potassium carefully, potassium replacement is commonly required.

6 Excessive urinary losses are most likely to occur after relief of obstruction or during the diuretic phase of ARF

7 Replacement should be according to urinary sodium losses

8 The treatment of adrenal insufficiency is described in Table 4.50

Table 4.9. Guide to quantity of sodium ions lost in a patient with sodium depletion

Body weight prior to illness (kg) = W
ECF (l) = F

ECF volume $(F) = W \times \dfrac{15}{10}$

Sodium deficit (mmol/l) = normal serum sodium − calculated serum sodium

Total sodium deficit (mmol/l) = $F \times$ sodium deficit (mmol/l)

Table 4.10. The management of water intoxication

Investigations
serum electrolytes, serum creatinine
Astrup analysis
BG
chest X-ray
analysis of urinary sodium

Management
assess level of consciousness—adequacy of airway
insert RAP line
insert urinary catheter and observe urine output

1 *Severe intoxication*. Semicomatose, twitching and/or convulsions. Ventilate if airway poor and/or hypoxic. Ventilation maintain PaO_2 around 10 kPa (75 mmHg) and $PaCO_2$ around 4.0 kPa (30 mmHg)
  • RAP 0-4 cmH$_2$O give 500 ml normal saline every 30 min until convulsions cease and/or Na$^+$ 130 mmol/l or more

180 *continued*

Table 4.10—*continued*

- slow down infusion if RAP >8 cms H_2O
- RAP normal (4-8 cm H_2O) give 100 ml twice normal saline (30 mmol Na^+/100 ml) every 20 min until convulsions cease and/or Na^+ is 130 mmol/l or more. Change to normal saline and slow down infusion rate if RAP >8 cm H_2O
- RAP high: suspect renal failure; exclude pulmonary oedema
- pulmonary oedema—intubate and ventilate
- oliguria—give 100 ml twice normal saline (over 20 min) and observe urine output
- if fluid challenge shows a hypervolaemic response (p. 105) and/or urine output <40 ml/h consider diuretics or renal dialysis
- metabolic acidosis if pH 7.20 or less and BD 10 or more, give 50 mmol sodium bicarbonate (50 ml 8.4%) over 20 min. Recheck acid base state 1 h after infusion stopped

2 *Moderate intoxication.* Drowsy response to simple commands, often twitching. Ventilation rarely required. Proceed as above

---

Table 4.11. Factors affecting potassium shifts between the intracellular and extracellular compartments

Changes in external balance

Alterations in K^+ intake

Sodium excess	Loss of K in urine	Se K ↓
Sodium deficiency	K comes out of the intracellular compartments	Se K ↑
Serum sodium deficiency	Increased urinary K loss	Se K↓
Acidosis	K comes out of the cell in exchange for hydrogen ions	Se K ↑
Alkalosis	K enters the cell in exchange for hydrogen ions	Se K ↓

Changes in cell metabolism

Cellular uptake of glucose	Se K ↓
Depletion of glycogen stores	Se K ↓
Protein anabilism	Se K ↓
Protein catabolism	Se K ↑
Intravascular haemolysis	Se K ↑
Hyperpyrexia	Se K ↑

continued

Table 4.11. — *continued*
Miscellaneous factors

Insulin	Se K ↓
Steroids	Se K ↓
Succinyl choline	Se K ↑
Thiazide diuretics	Se K ↓
Aldosterone antagonists	Se K ↑

Table 4.12. Factors producing a fall in total body potassium

Low potassium intake rarely produces K ↓ except during i.v. fluid therapy

Gastro-intestinal losses (see Table 4.7)
    Vomiting
    Nasogastric suction
    Ileus
    Biliary drainage
    Diarrhoea

Tumours
    Primary aldosteronism
    Cushing's syndrome

Renal losses
    Stress (see p. 143)
    Sodium overload
    Secondary aldosteronism
    Alkalosis
    Hypercalcaemia
    Previous renal tubular failure
    During recovery from ARF
    Drugs

Table 4.13. Treatment of hypokalaemia

1 Establish the cause (see previous table)
2 Analyse secretions and urine for potassium content
3 Assess renal function

continued

Table 4.13—*continued*

4 Stop all factors which may lower the serum potassium: i.v. dextrose solutions, insulin or digoxin therapy, sodium bicarbonate, diuretics

5 Do *not* hyperventilate the patient

6 Do *not* use sodium bicarbonate if the Se K is <3.2 mmol for the treatment of a metabolic acidosis

7 Check blood glucose, blood urea electrolytes, calcium magnesium levels if hypocalcaemia or hypomagnesaemia is a possibility

8 Assess the approximate quantity of K ions that have been lost (history analysis of secretions fluid balance) and attempt to replace ⅓ to ½ of the estimated losses within the first 24 h; to this must be added the continuing losses

9 Chronic depletion with no continuing losses replace orally

10 Acute severe potassium depletion (Se K <2.8 mmol/l) give potassium (as potassium chloride) in normal or 1/5 normal saline. Where fluid overload is suspected insert a RAP line (avoid too deep an insertion with excitation of the tricuspid valve). Rate of administration depends upon the clinical state of the patient.

Where respiratory paresis is present necessitating intubation and hand ventilation and/or serious cardiac dysrrhythmia, give 100 ml of 1/5 normal saline containing 40 mmol potassium chloride over 15-30 min. Tetany may develop during the infusion which reverses rapidly

Then replace as above, concentration depending on the circulating blood volume

Where there is anxiety about fluid overload infuse 40 mmol potassium chloride in 100 ml 1/5 normal saline every 2-4 h until Se K 3.0 mmol/l then slow down the infusion rate.

Normal saline may be used if the patient is Na depleted

Avoid fluid overload. Observe for onset of ARF and swing to hyperkalaemia

Se K should be checked 2 hourly, stopping the infusion 30 min

prior to taking the blood sample

Observe ECG—the appearance of the T wave is an indication to slow down infusion rate

In certain conditions (long term i.v. fluids, pancreatitis) calcium magnesium and phosphate ions may also require replacement

11 Moderate potassium depletion: Se K may be replaced more slowly, but is generally given i.v.

Table 4.14. Causes of potassium excess

Acute and acute on chronic renal failure

Metabolic or respiratory acidosis

Adrenal insufficiency	Addison's disease
	hypoaldosteronism

Hyperkalaemic periodic paralysis

Cell breakdown	hypercatabolic states
	acute intravascular haemolysis
	malignant hyperpyrexia

Iatrogenic	potassium sparing diuretics
	exogenous potassium
	massive transfusion of old blood
	succinyl choline

Table 4.15. Emergency treatment of acute hyperkalaemia

Drug	Dose	Onset of action	Duration	Comments
Calcium chloride	10% 0.45 mmol Ca^{2+}/ml 15-20 ml in 50 ml 1/5 normal saline Infuse over 5 min	min	<1h	Does not alter serum potassium Eliminates cardiotoxicity Necrotic to veins
Insulin and dextrose	50% dextrose (5 g CHO/ml) Infuse 25-50 g CHO with insulin 1 unit/4 g dextrose Give over 15-20 min	Min	Up to 4 h	Danger of hyperglycaemia—may require more insulin May be infused 4-6 hourly with appropriate insulin dosage
Exchange resin in sodium or calcium phase	50-60 g as a sorbitol retention enema or via Ryles tube	Approx. 30 min	4-6 h	Sodium overload with sodium phase resin Diarrhoea Has to be given via the gastro-intestinal tract

Table 4.16. Causes of acute hypocalcaemia

Acute pancreatitis

Hypoparathyroidism
  Post thyroidectomy
  Rarely idiopathic

Acute illness superimposed upon background calcium deficiency, vitamin D deficiency, or both
  Partial gastrectomy
  Intestinal disease including
    intestinal resections
    regional ileitis
    intestinal blind loop
    gluten enteropathy
  Obstructive jaundice

Chronic renal failure

Anticonvulsant therapy

Table 4.17. Mangement of acute hypocalcaemia

1 Identify the cause
2 Give i.v. calcium gluconate 10% (0.25 mmol Ca^2/ml) 10-20 ml over 10 min
3 Calcium losses continuing or tetany recurs give a calcium infusion 5-10 mmol Ca^2 every 4-12 h (calcium gluconate 10% 10 ml = 2.5 mmol Ca^2, calcium chloride 10% 10 ml = 4.5 mmol Ca^2)
4 Add calcium solution to 100 ml 1/5 normal saline and infuse to restore Se Ca to >2.0 mmol/l
5 *Always dilute* calcium solution, it is very necrotic on veins
6 Combination of hypocalcaemia and hyperkalaemia is particularly dangerous and may lead to cardiac arrest

Further management
1 Treat hypomagnesaemia (tetany does not respond to Ca^2 if hypomagnesaemia also present)
2 Vitamin D administration, oral or intravenous calcium supplements (Cohen 1978)

Table 4.18. Causes of hypercalcaemia

Malignancy
 multiple myelomatosis
 other haematological malignancies
 bony metastases
 humoral (no bony metastases)

Hyperparathyroidism
 primary
 associated with chronic renal failure

Vitamin D intoxication

Thyrotoxicosis

Addison's disease

Sarcoidosis

Immobilization

Renal failure acute during recovery phase

Table 4.19. General and specific therapy for acute hypercalcaemia

General
High fluid turnover rate
High sodium intake
Albumin infusion
Mannitol infusion

Treat concomitant metabolic deficiencies
 hypokalaemia
 hypomagnesaemia
Avoid the use of digitalis preparations

continued

Table 4.19—*continued*

Specific
Intravenous frusemide
Intravenous disodium hydrogen phosphate
Calcitonin

Therapeutic measures specific for certain causes of hypercalcaemia

Steroids
   vitamin D intoxication
   sarcoidosis
   malignant disease (occasionally effective)

Prostaglandin inhibitors (indomethacin, aspirin)
   solid malignancies

Mithramycin
   non-specific

Table 4.20. Causes of hypomagnesaemia

Deficient intake
   prolonged intravenous fluids without magnesium supplementation
   protein malnutrition

Decreased absorption
   malabsorption syndrome
   high calcium diet

Excessive urinary loss
   hyperaldosteronism primary or secondary
   renal tubular defects
   prolonged diuresis especially with thiazides

Excessive gastro-intestinal losses
   diarrhoea
   aspiration or fistula losses

Transfer from the extracellular fluid to other body compartments
   insulin therapy ($Mg^{2+} \rightarrow$ cell)
   following parathyroidectomy ($Mg^{2+} \rightarrow$ bone)
   acute pancreatitis (Mg^{2+} precipitate on peritoneum)

Table 4.21. Treatment of hypomagnesaemia

1 Find the cause (see previous table) and treat appropriately
2 Check calcium electrolytes and acid base state
3 Severe depletion (tetany or cardiac dysrrhythmia) give
10 mmol of magnesium sulphate (50% magnesium sulphate
2 mmol/ml) added to 50 ml of 1/5 normal saline and infuse
over 5-15 min. Follow with approximately 20 mmol magnesium
ions over 4 h
4 A mixed deficiency requires careful simultaneous infusion of
ionic mixtures. Suggested regime:

Calcium chloride 10 ml 10% (4.5 mmol Ca^{2+}) ⎫ in 100 ml
and potassium chloride 10 ml 15% (20 mmol K^+) ⎪ of 1/5
by separate infusion ⎬ normal
followed by ⎪ saline
magnesium sulphate 5 ml 50% (10 mmol Mg^{2+}) ⎭ in 100 ml
1/5 normal
saline

5 Infuse mixtures 2-6 hourly depending upon the level of
deficiency, whether losses are continuing, and based on
sequential biochemical and ECG monitoring

Table 4.22. Treatment of severe hypophosphataemia

1 Stop nutrition (glucose and amino acids) until serum phosphate is > 0.6 mmol/l
2 Intravenous preparation
Dipotassium hydrogen phosphate or monosodium phosphate
(100 mmol phosphate/l) if Se K > 5.0 mmol/l
Serum level < 0.4 mmol/l
3 Mix 10 mmol of phosphate with 100-200 ml 1/5 normal saline
High concentrations of dipotassium hydrogen phosphate are
necrotic on veins
4 Infuse 0.3 mmol of phosphate (as dipotassium hydrogen
phosphate)/kg BW over 2-4 h
5 Repeat the dose over the subsequent 4-6 hours and then
recheck serum phosphate
Serum level 0.41-0.7 mmol/l
6 Infuse the same dosage 12 hourly and check serum phosphate
after a total of 0.6 mmol/kg BW has been given
7 Observe ECG Se electrolytes, in particular Se K, Se calcium,
Se magnesium
8 Maintain a urine output of at least 40 ml/h

Table 4.23. Respiratory acid base disturbances: classification

Respiratory acidosis	Respiratory alkalosis
Pulmonary failure	Psychogenic hyperventilation
Neuromuscular failure	Hyperventilation secondary
Thoracic cage deformities	to pulmonary failure
Failure of the respiratory centre	Stimulation of the respiratory
	centre

Table 4.24. Metabolic acid base disturbances: classification

Metabolic alkalosis
Ingestion or infusion of alkali in excess of excreting ability
Inappropriate loss of acid
   Pyloric obstruction (renal and gastric losses)
   Renal losses
      potassium depletion
      chloride depletion
      hyperaldosteronism

Metabolic acidosis
High anion gap acidosis
Normal anion gap acidosis

Table 4.25. Physiological consequences of a metabolic acidosis

Pulmonary effect
   hyperventilation
Haemodynamic effects in severe metabolic acidosis
   fall in cardiac output
   cardiac dysrrhythmias
   arteriolar dilation (especially cerebral)
   venoconstriction

continued

Table 4.25—*continued*

Metabolic effects
  glycolysis decreased
  hepatic removal of lactate decreased
  extracellular potassium shift→Se K ↑
  increased urinary loss of Na^+ and K^+ with H_2O→ dehydration
  increased urinary loss of Ca^{2+} in chronic acidosis

Haematological effects
  acute acidosis—right shift of oxyHb dissociation curve
  (Bohr effect)
  chronic acidosis—return of oxyHb dissociation curve to normal
  position (2,3 DPG↓)
  leucocytosis

Table 4.26. Causes of a primary metabolic acidosis

Normal anion gap (5-12 mEq/l)	Increased anion gap (>12 mEq/l)
Diarrhoea	Diabetic ketoacidosis
Small bowel losses	Alcoholic ketoacidosis
Ureterosigmoid anastomosis	Lactic acidosis
Renal tubular acidosis	Intoxications
	salicylate
Excess administration of	methanol
ammonium chloride	paraldehyde
arginine monohydrochloride	ethylene glycol
	Renal failure
	Hepatic failure

4.7 Tables

Table 4.27. Treatment of a metabolic acidosis
(other than lactic acidosis)

1 A severe acidosis can generally be corrected by raising the standard bicarbonate to 5 mmol/l.

2 *Precautions Do not use bicarbonate* when Se K <3.5 mmol/l.
   Do not use in excess because of:
      sodium overload
      overcorrection resulting in adverse metabolic effects

3 Do not rely on hyperventilation for correction since it may continue for some time after pH is normal

4 Do not base therapy on the level of base deficit

5 Observe fluid balance and RAP in patients with renal or cardiac failure

6 Do not add any drugs to a sodium bicarbonate infusion

7 Rarely necessary to give sodium bicarbonate until pH 7.2 or less

8 Correct associated factors (volume depletion, hypoxia, hyperglycaemia)

9 Give sodium bicarbonate 50 mmol slowly i.v. as a bolus or infused in 1/5 normal saline over 30 min. Check pH 20 min later, if still <7.2 repeat dosage. Should pH not have improved after 100 mmol HCO_3 consider lactic acidosis (p.153)

10 Observe Se Na and K and ECG carefully. Start K infusion once Se K 3.5 mmol or less

11 Evidence of renal failure or left ventricular failure (LVF) or overload may be an indication for renal dialysis

Table 4.28. Classification of lactic acidosis

Type A lactic acidosis
   Shock, hypoxia

Type B lactic acidosis

Type B1	*Type B2*	*Type B3*
Common disorders	Drugs and toxins	Hereditary
Diabetes mellitus	Biguanides	e.g. glycogen storage
Renal failure	i.v. solutions	disease
Liver disease	fructose	Fructose 1.6 -
Infection	sorbitol	diphosphatase
Leukaemia	ethanol	deficiency
	Salicylates	
	Methanol	

Table 4.29. Conditions which predispose a patient to lactic acidosis

Underlying chronic renal or liver disease

Infection

Diabetes mellitus

Pancreatitis

Shock

Hyperventilation

Disseminated intravascular coagulation

Drugs
   phenformin
   fructose
   alcohol

Table 4.30. Treatment of lactic acidosis

1   Treat the underlying condition
2   Severe lactic acidosis suspected when aliquots of sodium bicarbonate (p. 192) fail to raise the pH above 7.2 or, after initial rise pH falls again
3   Insert a RAP line
4   Use 1/5 normal saline or PPF for volume replacement. Avoid normal saline. Maintain pH at 7.1 or more by a continuous bicarbonate infusion (generally 50 mmol bicarbonate in 100 ml 1/5 normal saline)
5   Rate regulated according to sequential pH levels. Commence at a rate of 50 mmol bicarbonate every 1-2 h
6   Observe urine output, serum potassium, RAP
7   Should RAP be >6 cm and urine output poor and or pH failing to improve, commence peritoneal dialysis
8   *Avoid* hypothermia, hypoxia, artificial ventilation (unless absolutely necessary) hypoglycaemia, hyperglycaemia, old blood
9   Artificial ventilation *if essential* ensure adequate CO and circulating blood volume and *hyperventilate* (cardiac output studies may be necessary since hyperventilation may reduce cardiac output and optimization of volume may require PCWP monitoring)
10   Consider   dextrose 50% (50g 4-6 hourly) with insulin if necessary to maintain blood glucose 6.0-10 mmol/l
    Anticoagulant therapy
11   Peritoneal dialysis indicated with hypotonic solution (p. 203) if serum sodium >152 mmol/l

Table 4.31. Factors, mechanism and treatment of primary metabolic alkalosis likely to be encountered in the critically ill

Aetiology	Mechanism	Urine chloride	Treatment
Chloride-responsive alkalosis			
Gastric aspirate or vomiting	Cl⁻ depletion	<10-20 mmol/l	Sodium chloride
Diuretic administration	Severe potassium depletion		Potassium chloride
Villous adenoma of colon			
Residual alkalosis following correction of hypercapnoea			Sodium chloride

Aetiology	Mechanism	Urine Chloride	Treatment
Chloride-resistant alkalosis			
Prolonged high dose administration of steroids	Increased distal tubular exchange of Na^+ for H^+ and K^+	>10-20 mmol/l	Stop steroids Potassium chloride
Chronic potassium depletion	Shift of K^+ from the cell in exchange with $H^+ \rightarrow$ intracellular acidosis		Potassium replacement
Rapid bicarbonate or lactate administration (in particular in renal failure)	HCO_3^- load exceeding renal excretion		Discontinue administration Consider arginine monohydrochloride
Citrate bladder irrigations			

Table 4.32. Normal values and porphyrin level changes in the porphyrias

	Urinary porphobilinogen 0-16 µmol/24 h	Urinary uroporphyrin 0-49 nmol/24 h	Urinary coproporphyrin 1-432 nmol/l 24 h	Faecal protoporphyrin 0-200 nmol/g dry wt	Faecal coproporphyrin 0-76 nmol/g dry wt
Normal levels					
Condition					
Acute intermittent porphyria	Raised — very high in attack	Usually raised	Sometimes raised	Sometimes raised	Sometimes raised
Porphyria variegata	Raised in attack	Sometimes raised	Sometimes raised	Raised	Raised
Hereditary coproporphyria	Raised only in attack	Sometimes raised in attack	Usually raised — always raised in attack	Usually normal	Raised

Table. 4.33. Drugs or factors which may aggravate or precipitate acute porphyria

Drugs
anticonvulsants of the hydantoin and succinimide group
barbiturates
chlordiazepoxide
glutethimide
griseofulvin
meprobamate
methyl dopa
sulphonamides
sulphonylureas

Factors
menstruation
decreased calorie intake
infection
alcohol excess

Table 4.34. Treatment of acute porphyria

1 Metabolic: Insert RAP line and correct metabolic abnormality.
   A low serum sodium may be due to the inappropriate release
   of ADH. Water intoxication is therefore a hazard. Use
   promazine for vomiting.
2 Haemodynamic management: Severe hypertension and an
   associated tachycardia consider the use of propranolol
   (1 mg i.v./min to a maximum of 10 mg stopping once the
   pulse rate <80/min)
   Consider the use of labetolol if there is peripheral vasoconstriction. Hypertension in the absence of tachycardia consider
   sedation alone (papaveretum)
   Do not use methyl dopa
3 Neurological management: Difficulty in swallowing, early
   evidence of bulbar involvement, rising $PaCO_2$, fall in tidal
   volume, an indication for intubation and ventilation. Use
   phenoperidine and diazepam or lorazepam for sedation on the
   ventilator. Fits, use paraldehyde, clonazepam or diazepam
   Do not use barbiturates or phenytoin
4 Nutrition:
   Give 250-400 g glucose daily. Monitor blood glucose carefully
   and give insulin if necessary
   Give 100-140 g protein daily, orally or i.v. as vamin glucose.
5 Skin: Avoid skin trauma. Avoid exposure to sunlight. Prick
   skin blisters and cover with paraffin gauze

Table 4.35. Characteristics of major disturbances on intracellular and extracellular volume and solute concentration in the presence of normal renal function

Type of disturbance	Volume			Osmolality		
	Extracellular	Intracellular	Intravascular	Serum	Urine	Serum sodium
Predominant water depletion (other than diabetes insipidus)	D	D	D	I	I	I
Water intoxication (other than inappropriate ADH secretion)	I	I	I	D	D	D
Acute salt intake	I	D	I	I	I	I

continued

Table 4.35—*continued*

Predominant salt loss	D	I	D	D	D	D
Acute sugar intake producing acute hyperglycaemia	I	D	I	I	—	N,D,I
Haemodilution e.g. CRF (chronic renal failure)					D generally	
Cardiac failure	I	I	N,D,I	D	N	D

D, decreased; I, increased; N, normal

4.7 Tables

Table 4.36. Factors producing the hyperosmolar syndrome

Predisposing factors
diabetes mellitus diagnosed or undiagnosed
uraemia particularly when acute
acute pancreatitis
stress in particular related to trauma and sepsis
patients undergoing renal dialysis

Precipitating factors
oral or intravenous glucose
low residence liquid diets

Drugs producing hyperglycaemia
corticosteroids
diazoxide

Drugs and fluids producing hypernatraemia
sodium bicarbonate
oral salt used as an emetic
sodium-containing antibiotics, e.g. carbenicillin
twice normal saline; normal saline used in the presence of dominant water depletion

Irrigating solutions
hypertonic dialysis solutions
lavage of the stomach, bowel or bladder with a hypertonic solution

Situations producing excessive water loss in relation to sodium
Diuretics
Burns
Fistula losses, severe diarrhoea
Starvation and dehydration
Situations producing acute uraemia e.g. acute intrinsic renal failure

Table 4.37. Treatment of the hyperosmolar syndrome of slow onset (serum osmolality < 350 mosmol/kg)

Predominant hyperglycaemia

1 Insulin soluble 12 units i.v. or i.m. stat then 8-12 units i.v. or i.m. hourly
2 Check BG Reflomat 1 hourly. BG 4 hourly
3 Stop insulin once BG 9 mmol/l or less
4 Water via the Ryles tube and/or i.v. ½ N or 1/5 N saline
5 Rate of fluid administration approximately 1 l 4-hourly for 24 h—increase initial rate if there is evidence of severe dehydration
6 Observe for hypokalaemia, onset of ARF fluid overload or DIC

Predominant hypernatraemia

1 Fluids as above
2 Observe for hyperglycaemia, hypokalaemia, onset of ARF or CCF
3 *Do not give diuretics*
4 *Dialyse peritoneally* with a hypotonic dialysate should the basic deficit be > 10 or pH 7.1 or less, or there is evidence of ARF
5 Dialysis solution—either Hartmann's solution if Se K⁺ normal and BG 6 mmol/l or greater or 1 l Hartmann's solution followed by 500 ml 1.3% dialaflex solution

Table 4.38. Summary of treatment of the hyperosmolar syndrome related predominantly to hypernatraemia

Investigations

1 On admission:
• BU electrolytes
• BG serum osmolality
• Blood gases, acid base state
• Hb, PCV, clotting indices
  Repeat 2-4 hourly
2 With excessive oral ingestion of sodium ions introduce a Ryles tube, measure the volume and the sodium concentration. Estimate the anticipated rise in Se Na (p. 156)
3 Eliminate the sodium source

4.0 Specific problems

4.7 Tables

Intravenous fluids
1 Insert a RAP line and infuse up to a normal level with 1/5 normal saline. Maintain RAP at a normal level and encourage a high urine flow with 1 l of 1/5 normal saline i.v. 3-4 hourly. Slow down rate if RAP >8 cm H_2O.
2 ECG monitoring and sequential observation of Se K and BG essential.
3 *Do not* use sodium bicarbonate.

Convulsions
1 i.v. phenytoin
2 i.m. paraldehyde
3 Should a benzodiazepine be used, observe for respiratory depression
4 *Do not* use chlormethiazole (sodium content 30-34 mmol/l)

Intravascular haemolysis
1 Give whole blood if Hct 30% or less
2 Ventilation indicated under the following circumstances
   • continuous twitching or convulsions
   • inadequate airway maintenance
   • inadequate ventilation
   • increasing metabolic acidosis
   • pulmonary oedema
   • rising $PaCO_2$ or PaO_2 8.7 kPa (65 mmHg) or less
3 Catheterize; maintain urine output at >60 ml/h. If urine output <40 ml/h in the presence of a normal RAP suspect renal failure. Check U/P osmolality ratio—if <1.2—commence renal dialysis
4 Insulin; if BG 10 mmol/l or more (see Table 4.42)
5 Lumbar puncture indications:
   • deterioration in level of consciousness
   • localizing neurological signs
   • neck stiffness
6 Renal dialysis indicated:
   • following oral ingestion anticipated Na^+ rise >20 mmol/l
   • presence of renal failure
   • presence of fluid overload
7 Solution see previous table on p. 203
8 Rate 500 ml every 30 min continuous recycling, add K to the dialysate if necessary

Table 4.39. Total body water (l) in relation to age and sex

Age	Male	Female
10-18	59	57
18-40	61	51
40-60	55	47
>60	52	46

Modified from Edelman & Liebman (1959)

Table 4.40. Summary of treatment of the hyperosmolar syndrome due to hyperglycaemia
(unrelated to diabetes mellitus)

1 Insulin actrapid
   - 16 units i.v. BG >18 mmol/l
   - 12 units i.v. 12-17.9 mmol/l
2 Then continue Actrapid insulin 8 units hourly until BG = 10.0 mmol or less
3 This may be given as a continuous infusion (in haemaccel) or as i.v. boluses
4 If BG not decreasing inc. hourly dosage to 12 units i.v.
5 i.v. fluids:
   - give 1/5 normal saline or normal saline according to Se sodium (*do not give* normal saline if Se Na >140 mmol/l)
   - Rate according to table on p. 204
6 *Do not* give sodium bicarbonate unless pH 7.1 or less, then 50 mmol *at the most*
7 Sodium bicarbonate contraindicated if Se osmolality >350 mosmol/kg.
8 Catheterize; see table on p. 204
9 Serial investigations; see Table 4.38
10 Observe for fall in serum sodium, onset of fluid overload, and ARF or DIC

Table 4.41. Differential diagnosis of hyperosmolar states with diabetes mellitus

	Dehydration	Ketosis	Base deficit	Ventilation	Insulin
DKA diabetic ketoacidosis	+++	+++	+++	+++	+++
NKA Non-ketotic hyperglycaemia	+++	+ → 0	+ → 0	+	++
DM and lactic acidosis	+	Variable	++	++	Variable

4.0 Specific problems

4.7 Tables

Table 4.42. Management of diabetic ketoacidosis

1 On admission check:
   - BG serum osmolality
   - BU electrolytes
   - blood gases, acid base state
   - Hb, PCV, WBC and differential
   - clotting factors
2 Action
   - insert 2 i.v. drips (one for insulin and i.v. drugs, the other for volume and metabolic correction)
   - insert RAP line, record every 15 min initially
   - catheterize—record hourly urine volume
   - insert a Ryles tube—aspirate to dryness, put down 15 ml sodium citrate 0.3 M
3 i.v. fluids:
   - BP SP < 100 mmHg give PPF
   - BP SP > 100 mmHg, serum sodium < 145 mmol/l pH > 7.1 give normal saline
   - BP SP > 100 mmHg, serum sodium > 145 mmol/l—give 1/5 normal saline
   - BP SP > 100 mmHg, pH 7.1 or less, give 1/5 normal saline and 50 mmol aliquots of sodium bicarbonate (100 ml 1/5 normal saline + 50 mmol sodium bicarbonate infused over 20-30 min
   - infuse appropriate fluid 500 ml every 15 min until the RAP 2-4 cm H_2O and urine output > 40 ml/h
   - subsequent fluid to be given dependent on serum sodium and blood pH. Once RAP restored generally best to change to 1/5 normal saline. 500 ml i.v. every 2-4 h
4 i.v. potassium 10-20 mmol/hour once Se K is 3.5 mmol/l or less
5 Insulin Actrapid
   - 16 units i.v. BG > 18 mmol/l
   - 12 units i.v. BG 12-17.9 mmol/l
     Then continue Actrapid insulin 8 units i.v. hourly until BG 10.0 mmol/l or less
     If BG not decreasing, increase hourly dose to 12 units
6 Search for factors precipitating DKA and treat
7 Ventilation consider if $PaO_2 < 9.3$ kPa (70 mmHg) or $PaCO_2 > 8.0$ kPa (60 mmHg)
   Should ventilation be indicated—ensure maintenance of haemodynamic state. Hyperventilate initially in order to compensate for metabolic acidosis

8   Dialysis—rarely indicated:
   * indicated if evidence of ARF
   * suspect if urine output <40 ml/h in spite of restoration of blood volume
9   Observe for vomiting complicated by aspiration, metabolic mismanagement (Se sodium ↑ Se K ↓), and DIC
10   Should level of consciousness not improve over 6 h, consider lumbar puncture
11   Observe for lactic acidosis complicating DKA
12   Subsequent management:
   * check BG hourly
   * insulin according to BG
   * urea electrolytes 2-4 hourly.
   * blood gases, acid base state ½-4 hourly (depending upon initial results)

Table 4.43. Summary of treatment of severe diabetic non-ketotic hyperglycaemia

1   i.v. fluids: Set up RAP
   * RAP <2 cm H_2O. Serum Na^+ >150 mmol/l
     1/5 N saline—1 l over 1 h then 1 l 2-hourly until RAP >4
   * RAP <2 cm H_2O. Serum Na^+ <150 mmol/l
     ½ N saline—1 litre over 1 h then 1/5 N saline as above.
   * RAP 4-12 cm H_2O
     1/5 N saline approx 1 litre 4-hourly
   * RAP >12 cm H_2O. No clinical or X-ray evidence of pulmonary oedema
     1/5 N saline as a fluid challenge (see fig. on p. 105) until RAP >12 cm then 1 l approx. 8-hourly
   * RAP >12 cm H_2O and evidence of LV overload, proceed to—
2   Hypotonic peritoneal dialysis: rate approx. 500 ml every 30 min. Observe serum K and BG. Maintain RAP 4-10 cm H_2O with i.v. 1/5 N saline
3   Insulin Actrapid: BG <25 mmol/l 16 units i.m. or i.v. stat. then 4 units i.v. or i.m. hourly, BG >25 mmol/l 20 units i.m. or i.v. stat. then 8 units i.v. or i.m. hourly. Observe BG and Se K. Stop insulin when BG 10 mmol or less
4   Catheterize: Check U/P osmolality ratio. Urine output <40 ml/h once RAP normal and/or U/P osmolality rate 1.2 or less, start peritoneal dialysis

continued

Table 4.43—*continued*

5   Ryles tube: If gastric retention, aspirate and put down 15 ml 0.3 M sodium citrate. Commence water 20 ml hourly—once able to absorb, slow down i.v. infusion

6   Potassium: Once urine output >40 ml/h give potassium at a rate of approx. 10-16 mmol/h (according to serum K^+)

7   Acidosis: *Do not* use sodium bicarbonate if serum Na >150 mmol/l. *Do not* give >50 mmol i.v. Dialyse if Se Na >150 mmol pH <7.1 or BD >15

8   Observe for vascular complications, infections, onset of renal failure, deterioration of level of consciousness with respiratory depression, hypokalaemia, hypoglycaemia

9   Ventilation: consider if gets respiratory depression, inadequate respiratory compensation for metabolic acidosis, convulsions uncontrolled with phenytoin sodium

10   Check BG (Reflomat) hourly. BG, urea, electrolytes, Astrup 2-4 hourly. Clotting factors—evidence of DIC and clinical evidence of vascular occlusion, consider low dose of heparin

Table 4.44. Myxoedema coma: precipitating factors

Infection

Myocardial infarction

Cerebrovascular accident

Trauma

Drugs
   benzodiazepines
   barbiturates
   chlorpromazine

Table 4.45. Myxoedema coma: manifestations

Clinical
    hypothyroid appearance
    stuporose
    hypothermia is common
    bradycardia
    slowed reflexes
    oedema and cardiac failure common
    evidence of precipitating factor

Biochemical
    Se Na ↓ (dilutional) BG often ↓
    Se cholesterol ↑
    pH often ↓ $PaCO_2$ ↑ PaO_2 ↓
    macrocytosis Hb generally ↓
    T_3T_4 ↓ (common in cold old people)
    TSH ↑ (diagnostic)

Table 4.46. Myxoedema coma: treatment

Rewarming
1   Place patient on an electrically heated warming blanket
2   Wrap in a space blanket
3   Record core temperature
4   Rewarm to core temperature of 33°C then turn off electric blanket and leave under space blanket
5   Warm all fluids given i.v. or intragastrically

Respiration and maintenance of blood gases
1   Check blood gases. Correct levels according to core temperature
2   Adjust oxygen via face mask in order to avoid CO_2 narcosis
3   Maintain end tidal CO_2 at 9.0 kPa or less
4   Insert a RAP line, a high fixed level with little swing suggests tamponade, pericardial tap may be necessary
5   Maintain RAP low normal 2-6 cm H_2O. Use PPF for volume replacement
6   Ventilate if PaO_2 <7.0 kPa. Use minimum of sedation and a muscle relaxant. Adjust ventilation to perfusion (p. 42)

continued

Table 4.46—*continued*

7 Ventilation may also be indicated in
 • severe cardiac failure
 • pulmonary sepsis
8 Ventilator weaning is often difficult, tracheostomy is commonly indicated

Control of electrolyte imbalance
1 Hyponatraemia generally dilutional, *do not give* crystalloid for volume replacement use PPF
2 Careful fluid balance *do not* overload, adjust according to RAP and urine output (catheterize if necessary)
3 Give 150-200 g carbohydrate daily as 50% dextrose i.v. or caloreen via Ryles tube.
4 *Do not* start oral feed until sure of airway
5 Observe for fluctuations in BG, BG >12.0 mmol/l give Actrapid insulin 4 units i.v. hourly prn. (these patients are very sensitive to insulin)

Treatment of cardiac complications
1 *Do not* treat bradycardia if perfusion adequate
2 If perfusion poor use *very low* doses of isoprenaline to achieve a SP of 80 mm
3 Do not use inotropes if tamponade present
4 Use thiazide diuretics with care, hypokalaemia common

Hormone replacement
1 Avoid high doses, oral absorption erratic therefore often necessary to give intravenously as T_3 10 μg i.v. twice daily for 3 days increasing to 40 μg daily. Once oral absorption secure give T_4
2 Hydrocortisone 100 mg i.v. stat then i.v. 8 hourly for four to six doses

Treatment of infection
1 Do not give prophylactic antibiotics
2 Creatinine clearance often low so therefore regulate drug therapy accordingly (p. 20)

4.0 Specific problems

Table 4.47. Thyroid crisis: manifestations

Sinus tachycardia cardiac dysrhythmias including VF

Cardiac failure

Pyrexia generally $> 38^{\circ}C$

Tremor

Sweating and hyperventilation

Neuropsychiatric manifestations
  extreme agitation
  occasionally apathy
  manic psychosis
  extreme confusion

Biochemical T_3 T_4 ↑. Often Na and water depleted

Table 4.48. Thyroid crisis: treatment

Take blood levels for T_3 and T_4

Reduction of oxygen demands
1 PaO_2 < 6.7 kPa, intubate and ventilate
2 High levels of sedatives are required, best to intubate using diazepam (20-30 mg i.v.) plus a muscle relaxant (pancuronium). *Do not* use suxamethonium
3 Continue sedation with diazepam and a background of i.m. chlorpromazine 25-50 mg 6 hourly
4 Measure core temperature and cool to $33^{\circ}C$
5 Use a cold water blanket; cold fluids dripped into the stomach; cooled i.v. fluids; sheet soaked in methylated spirits

Metabolic correction
1 Insert RAP line, restore RAP to 4 cm H_2O with PPF
2 Monitor BG, give insulin if BG > 12.0 mmol/l
3 Give 50 mmol sod. bicarbonate i.v. if pH < 7.1 and repeat if necessary (see p. 194 lactic acidosis)
4 Give 100 ml of 50% dextrose i.v. 6 hourly (insulin if necessary)
5 Check Se Ca Mg; hypercalcaemia rarely requires specific treatment

continued

Table 4.48 — *continued*

6 Digoxin if elderly and in AF, 0.5 mg titrated i.v. *slowly* then 0.5 mg i.m.

7 Cardiovert if patient in VT or VF

8 Propranolol in all cases unless a known asthmatic, has bronchospasm or in gross cardiac failure
  Give 5-15 mg titrated intravenously *slowly* (observe for bronchospasm myocardial depression, sudden bradycardia) then continuous infusion 5-15 mg i.v. 4 hourly

9 Presence of bronchospasm cardiac failure titrate i.v. *very slowly practolol* 5-10 i.v. 4 hourly

Specific therapy

1 Potassium iodide 200 mg i.v. over 15 min followed by Lugols iodine 10 drops 6 hourly via the Ryles tube

2 Propyl thiouracil 150 mg via Ryles tube 6 hourly

Additional therapy

1 Observe for postoperative complications in the patient with a recent operative procedure including hypocalcaemia post thyroidectomy

2 It is generally recommended that hydrocortisone should be given 100 mg i.v. stat then i.v. 8 hourly for 6 doses

Table 4.49. Addisonian crisis: manifestations

Abdominal pain and vomiting

Anorexia

Weakness

Pigmentation

Hypothermia and hypoglycaemia may be present

Hypotension

Dehydration

Biochemistry
  Se Na ↓ K ↑ BG ↓
  Basal cortisol ↓ ACTH ↑
  (short synacthin stimulation often not diagnostic)

Table 4.50. Addisonian crisis: treatment

Treat precipitating factor

Restoration of circulating blood volume: correction of metabolic imbalance

1 Insert RAP line
2 Restore circulating blood volume with normal saline, or if severely shocked and/or hypoalbuminaemia suspected, PPF
3 Observe urine output and Se K
4 Correct hypoglycaemia with intravenous dextrose 50%, insulin may be required following hormonal replacement

Hormonal replacement

1 Hydrocortisone 200 mg i.v. stat then 100 mg i.v. 6 hourly. In the presence of severe hyponatraemia give aldosterone 1 mg i.v.
2 Stabilize over the subsequent 3-4 days on oral cortisone acetate and 9d fluorohydrocortisone

Table 4.51. Treatment of hypercortisolism

Metabolic care

1 Correct hypokalaemia either by i.v. or oral potassium

Hormonal management

1 Hydrocortisone 20 mg 8 hourly for 3 doses, followed by metyrapone 500 mg t.i.d. increasing to 1.0 g t.i.d. if response is inadequate
2 Continue oral hydrocortisone
3 In spite of hydrocortisone observe for hypoadrenalism
4 Once acute crisis over investigate

Table 4.52. α- and β-adrenergic receptors: effects mediated by the two types of receptor

α-receptor	β-receptor
Vasoconstriction of all vascular beds, especially skin	Vasodilation of all vascular beds especially skeletal muscle
Constriction of: • nictitating membrane: • dilator pupillae • orbital smooth muscle	Relaxation of intestinal smooth muscle and bronchial smooth muscle
Relaxation of intestinal smooth muscle	Positive inotropic effect of heart muscle
	Positive chronotropic responses of heart muscle

Antagonists

Phentolamine Phenoxybenzamine	β-blockers (propranolol)

Mixed antagonism

$\alpha\ \beta$ blockade	labetolol

Table 4.53. Treatment of acute manifestations secondary to phaeochromocytoma

1 *Sequence of treatment is important*
2 *Provocation tests are an absolute contraindication* e.g. hypertensive response to abdominal palpation or histamine
3 Phentolamine test use with care, α-blockade may produce sudden hypovolaemic shock

Procedure

1 Insert a RAP line, be prepared to volume top up with PPF after α-blockade
2 Observe ECG. VF is common and ventricular dysrhythmias

continued

Table 4.53—*continued*

3 Record urine output. Peripheral and core temperature
4 Should myocardial failure be a problem consider PCWP monitoring (insertion of catheter hazardous because of precipitating a dysrhythmia)

Extreme hypertension
1 Phentolamine 2.5-5.0 mg i.v. as a bolus (lasts 5-10 min) Continue with intermittent bolus injections or regulate as an infusion, 1 mg/ml of 1/5 N saline adjust to maintain SP < 160 mmHg (0.5-2 mg/min). Observe for hypovolaemia, top up with PPF
2 Best to avoid *phenoxybenzamine* as an emergency because of prolonged activity; give orally once crisis is over

Tachycardia
1 This may be 'unleashed' as a result of phentolamine. Should hypertension be present always use phentolamine first
2 Propranolol: 1-5 mg i.v. until pulse rate < 120/min. Titrate slowly as patient may be very sensitive. Continue as an infusion 5-10 mg 4-8 hourly
3 Practolol: use where cardiac failure is suspected or present instead of propranolol as an intermittent bolus injection 5-10 mg.

Congestive cardiac failure and phaeochromocytoma
1 Very difficult to manage
2 Sedation and ventilation often advisable before using drugs
3 Cardiac failure may take weeks to resolve

Operative management
Described by Wright (1978)

Table 4.54. Hypopituitary coma: manifestations

Clinical
Patient may have soft pale skin, no body hair
Hypothermia
Hypotension
Acute pituitary infarction may arise during the course of:
• acromegaly
• prolactinoma

continued

Table 4.54—*continued*

- Cushing's syndrome, Nelson's syndrome
- non-functioning tumour

In these circumstances—headache, ophthalmoplegia common.

Biochemical

BG ↓

Na ↓ (dilutional)

T_4, cortisol, ACTH, TSH all low

X-ray of pituitary fossa may be abnormal

Table 4.55. Hypopituitary coma: treatment

General

1 Insert RAP line. *Do not fluid overload*
2 May require modest quantities of normal saline
3 Give dextrose 50% 100 ml i.v. 6 hourly, observe Se K

Hormonal

1 Hydrocortisone 200 mg i.v. stat then 100 mg i.v. 6 hourly
2 Start T_3 or T_4 24 h later

Table 4.56. Causes of diabetes insipidus and primary polydipsia

---

Cranial diabetes insipidus (CDI)

Familial

Acquired

- idiopathic
- head injury, neurosurgery
- tumours
- granulomata (sarcoidosis, tuberculosis, histiocytosis)
- infections (encephalitis meningitis)
- vascular (haemorrhage, sickle cell anaemia, aneurysms)

Nephrogenic diabetes insipidus (NDI)

Familial

Acquired

- metabolic Ca ↑ K ↓
- post-obstructive uropathy
- infections (pyelonephritis)
- toxic (lithium)
- osmotic effect (glucose)
- chronic renal disease

Primary polydipsia

Generally psychotic states

Table 4.57. Treatment of diabetes insipidus

Cranial diabetes insipidus
1 Mild (urine loss 2-4 l daily) — increase fluid intake
2 Moderate to severe:
 • may present with severe water depletion
 • fluid volume replace with 5% dextrose
 • use desmopressin by i.m. or i.v. injection 1-4 μg daily until able to take intranasally
 • prevent water intoxication, adjust dosage to maintain urine output around 2 l daily
 • *Do not* restrict oral fluids

Nephrogenic diabetes insipidus
1 Correct any underlying abnormality
2 Thiazide diuretics may be helpful
3 *Do not* restrict oral fluids

Table 4.58. Causes of meningitis according to age

Children <4 yr
 Haemophilus influenzae
 Neisseria meningitidis
 Streptococcus pneumoniae

Children 4 yr-adulthood
 Neisseria meningitidis
 Streptococcus pneumoniae

Other rarer causes
 Cryptococcus neoformans
 Listeria monocytogenes
 Pseudomonas aeruginosa
 Staphylococcus aureus
 Escherichia coli

Table 4.59. Treatment of purulent meningitis

1 When suspected—lumbar puncture, unless there are focal signs then arrange an urgent CAT scan
2 Antibiotics based on organisms seen in CSF treat specifically if possible
3 Seriously ill
   - intrathecal penicillin (special intrathecal preparation) 10 000 units benzyl penicillin
   - penicillin soluble 2 mega units i.v. 2 hourly
   - chloramphenicol 1.0 g i.v. 6 hourly

Supportive care

1 Observe core temperature, temperature $>40°C$ cool
2 Insert RAP line—restore circulating volume
3 Meningococcal ⎫ meningitis are often associated with cir-
   Pneumococcal ⎭ culatory collapse and DIC
4 Treat convulsions should they arise
5 Observe for CDI or Na ↓ due to inappropriate secretion of ADH
6 Localizing signs are an indication for a CAT scan

Table 4.60. Factors which may precipitate status epilepticus in a known epileptic

Drugs
   omission
   subtherapeutic
Stress and relaxation
Hypoglycaemia
   in diabetics
   preprandial
Alcohol
Menstruation
Pregnancy
Reflex
   stroboscopic activation
   sudden sound

Table 4.61. Range of blood levels in anticonvulsant therapy

| Anticonvulsant | Therapeutic range | | Toxic level |
	μmol/l	(μg/ml)	μmol/l
Carbamazepine	17-42	(4-10)	> 42
Ethosuximide	285-850	(40-120)	>859
Phenobarbitone	65-170	(15-40)	>170
Phenytoin	40-100	(10-25)	>100
Sodium valproate	350-700	(50-100)	>700

Table 4.62. Treatment of status epilepticus

Control of seizures
Drugs which may be used:
Diazepam 5-20 mg titrated slowly i.v.
Clonazepam 0.5-1.0 mg titrated slowly i.v.
    Observe the airway and adequacy of ventilation
Paraldehyde 5-10 ml i.m.
Paraldehyde 4-5 ml i.v.
    Necrotic on veins and injection sites
Chlormethiazole hemisucinate 0.8% solution, i.v. infusion. Infuse rapidly until status controlled then maintain at 60-90 ml/h (480-720 mg/h)
    Necrotic on veins, may produce respiratory depression
Phenytoin sodium up to 250 mg by slow i.v. injection rate not >50 mg/min
    Poorly absorbed i.m.
Author's preference:
Diazepam titrated slowly i.v.
Depression of subsequent seizures with i.v. heminevrin or i.m. paraldehyde
If previously on phenytoin give equivalent dosage down Ryles tube or i.v. 8 hourly
Supportive care
1 Treat any associated infection
2 Insert a RAP line, restore circulating volume and correct any metabolic imbalance
Ventilation
1 Indicated in severe status epilepticus (pulse rate >140/min)

continued

Table 4.62—*continued*

hypoxia pH <7.3) when the airway is at risk, when the patient is pregnant and PaO_2 <9.0 kPa
2   During ventilation sedate heavily for at least 24 h with:
  • diazepam 10 mg i.m. 4 hourly for 6 doses
  • i.v. heminevrin
3   Do not extubate until fever settled and pulse rate <110/min

Table 4.63. Treatment of acute severe idiopathic polyneuritis

1   Insert RAP line and maintain adequate circulating blood volume
2   Monitor pulse, skin core temperature differential and arterial blood pressure continuously
3   Observe airway control, ability to cough and swallow, respiratory rate and respiratory excursion
4   Record peak flow FVC hourly to 2 hourly
5   Observe PaO_2, $PaCO_2$
6   Monitor hourly urine output

Ventilate
1   Intubate and ventilate if:
  • patient unable to cough or maintain airway
  • falling FVC rising respiratory rate
  • rising $PaCO_2$
2   Ventilate early if there is evidence of infection, lung collapse or aspiration
3   Once intubated and ventilated perform tracheostomy early and continue to ventilate with background tranquillization e.g. diazepam

Management of autonomic complications
1   May require nursing flat in order to maintain adequate SP
2   Bradycardia or asystole with tracheal suction pre-medicate with atropine
3   Asystolic arrest often responds to patient stimulation and a blow on the lower sternum
4   Pulse rate extremely variable, avoid adrenergic agents and/or β-blockers. Numerous ventricular extrasystoles use minimal dose of i.v. lignocaine
5   Excessive sweating may require high volume fluid replacement
6   Uncontrollable diarrhoea—do not feed orally, may be helped with kaolin and morphine mixture 10 ml 3-8 hourly

7 Infection treat when it arises, *do not* use prophylactic antibiotics
8 Supportive care is extremely important including:
   - skin care
   - physiotherapy
   - urinary drainage
   - routine antacid therapy
   - prophylactic anticoagulant therapy as subcutaneous heparin 5000 units 8 hourly
9 Steroids—no evidence that they are of value
10 Plasmapheresis of no proven value to date

Table 4.64. Myasthenia gravis: treatment of a myasthenic crisis

Ventilation and airway control

1 Should ventilation be indicated because of adverse lung pathology or systemic disease. *Omit* anticholinergics and *do not* use muscle relaxants. Adequate sedation and analgesia is *absolutely essential*
2 When reversal is indicated, *commence* neostigmine methyl sulphate 1 mg (equivalent to 15 mg orally) i.m. 8 hourly increasing the frequency of the dose to 3 hourly if necessary. The requirement for the next dose should be assessed according to the forced vital capacity (FVC < 1.5 l) and large pupils. *Do not* use atropine in the first instance. Pupils <3 mm diameter suggests excess anticholinergic

Non ventilated critically ill patient

1 Perform an edrophonium test (see p. 162) if positive commence neostigmine methyl sulphate 1 mg i.m. and repeat the dose as above
2 Once patient able to absorb orally pyridostigmine bromide is often the preferred background anticholinergic using neostigmine as a 'booster'
3 Obtain a neurological opinion as soon as possible for subsequent and additional treatment

Table 4.65. Myasthenia gravis: treatment of a cholinergic crisis

1 Ventilation and airway control. Intubate and ventilate. Stop all anticholinergics
2 Observe for improvement in muscle power, VC and enlargement of pupils
3 Once vital capacity >1.5 l pupils >3 mm diameter commence anticholinergic in half the preceeding dosage i.m. in the first instance
4 Equivalent dosages of anticholinergics:
   • neostigmine methyl sulphate 15 mg orally or 1 mg i.m.
   • pyridostigmine bromide   60 mg orally or 1 mg i.m.
   • neostigmine methyl sulphate 15 mg orally has an equivalent activity to pyridostigmine bromide 60 mg orally

Table 4.66. Management of massive gastro-intestinal haemorrhage

1 Admit to ITU
2 Insert RAP line ensure at least two other i.v. lines available
3 Take blood for clotting factors
   • U & E, Hb, Hct,
   • astrop analysis
4 Volume replace according to Table 3.5 on p. 116
5 With volume replacement ensure that labile clotting factors are replaced observe for thrombocytopenia
6 Pass a Ryles tube aspirate hourly
7 Use routine antacid therapy 2 hourly
8 Consider the use of i.v. cimetidine
9 Once volume replacement under control and bleeding less brisk (falling pulse rate, steady blood pressure and RAP) arrange for endoscopy to establish bleeding source
10 Treatment according to bleeding source:
   • oesophageal varices see p. 56
   • Mallory Weiss—generally operate
   • gastric ulcer—operate if haemorrhage continues
   • duodenal ulcer—operate if repeated haemorrhage (post-operative complications $>$ gastric ulcer)

continued

Table 4.66—*continued*

- acute gastritis ⎫ remove any cause (asprin, anti-
- multiple erosions ⎬ inflammatory agents, steroids) give
                    cimetidine and antacids; avoid surgery if
                    at all possible

- Lower-gastro-
  intestinal   ⎫ sigmoidoscopy; avoid if possible any
  haemorrhage   ⎬ operation before definitive diagnosis
  (red blood P/R) ⎭ made

11 Gastrointestinal haemorrhage source not found by the above measures. Exclude hereditary telangiectasia. Should bleeding be at a rate >2 ml/min consider angiography. Emergency barium meal.

12 Timing of operation. Indications may vary from one centre to another. Operate earlier in patients >50 years. Reasonable indications are:
- whole blood transfusion >2500 ml first 24 h
- whole blood transfusion >1500 ml second 24 h
- rebleeding after 24 h of vigorous medical therapy

13 Preparation for operation. Ensure all clotting factors replaced, following massive haemorrhage give four packs of FFP pre-operatively. Platelet count <60 000/mm³ give four packs of FFP pre-operatively, four packs during and four packs postoperatively. Correct all metabolic deficits. In the critically ill ventilate postoperatively.

Table 4.67. Management of a patient presenting with acute diarrhoea

1 Set up an infusion, insert a RAP line
2 Check Se electrolytes, Astrup analysis, BG clotting factors, Ca^{2+} Mg^{2+} studies, blood cultures where sepsis is suspected, and stools — for culture or analysis for amoebae, helminths, histology
3 If severe shock present, replace circulating volume with PPF. Massive diarrhoea often associated with acute Ca^{2+} Mg^{2+} depletion, replace if necessary (pp. 186 and 189)
4 Establish diagnosis:
   • sigmoidoscopy
   • urgent barium meal/enema if necessary
5 Exclude any surgically correctable lesion or associated complication, e.g. perforation

Table 4.68. Management of acute severe ulcerative colitis

1 Proceed according to Table 4.67
2 Stop all fluids orally
3 Give blood if Hb <10.0 g/dl establish parenteral nutrition after metabolic correction
4 Give vitamin supplements
5 Commence prednisolone phosphate 60-80 mg i.v. daily and hydrocortisone enema (100 ml volume) 100 mg b.d.
6 Metronidazole 0.5 g i.v. 8 hourly
7 Observe metabolic state carefully. PPF one to two bottles daily to maintain Se albumin >30 g/l
8 Surgery is indicated if:
   • no improvement in condition after 5 days therapy
   • toxic dilatation of the colon not responding to 24 h medical treatment
   • suspected perforation
   • obstruction with suspected carcinoma or stricture formation

4.0 Specific problems

4.7 Tables

Table 4.69. Management of acute severe Crohn's disease

1 Proceed according to Table 4.67
2 Stop all fluids orally
3 Proceed according to Table 4.68, points 3-7 inclusive
4 Surgery may be indicated:
   - perforation suspected
   - evidence of severe systemic sepsis
   - obstruction
   - failure to respond to medical management with evidence of increasing 'toxemia' (generally secondary to systemic sepsis and localized perforation)

Table 4.70. Acute pancreatitis: indications for admission to an ITU

Clinical indications
   Shock
   Sepsis
   Haemorrhage
   Pancreatic encephalopathy
   Severe pain

Biochemical indications
   Electrolyte imbalance
   Hypoxia
   Metabolic acidosis
   Methaemalbuminaemia (MHA)

Haematological indications
   Anaemia
   High white cell count
   Haemorrhagic diathesis

4.0 Specific problems

4.7 Tables

Table 4.71. The acute early complications relating to pancreatitis

Hypotension
- hypovolaemic
- cardiac
- septic

Electrolyte imbalance
- sodium depletion
- potassium depletion
- hypocalcaemia
- hypomagnesaemia

Acid base imbalance
- metabolic alkalosis { hypokalaemia / vomiting
- metabolic acidosis { poor peripheral perfusion
- respiratory acidosis { carbondioxide retention / respiratory failure

Glucose intolerance

Pulmonary failure

Renal failure

Hepatic failure

Haematological complications

Table 4.72. Treatment of the early acute phase of pancreatitis

1 Insert RAP: restore circulating volume with PPF or, in the presence of anaemia and bleeding, blood
2 Check
   • BU electrolytes, BG, calcium magnesium, Se albumin
   • Astrup
   • U/P osmolality ratio
   • HB, WBC and diff. PCV
   • clotting factors
   • electrolyte analysis of intestinal losses if severe
3 Observe
   • fluid losses
   • urine output
   • ECG
   • respiratory state
4 Correct any *metabolic deficit*
5 Correct any *respiratory defect* if possible
   $PaO_2 < 10.0$ kPa (75 mmHg) oxygen via face mask
   Artificially ventilate if
   • PaO_2 fails to rise above 10.0 kPa (75 mmHg)
   • evidence of pulmonary aspiration
   • due for surgery
6 Check renal function evidence of acute renal failure, commence dextrose/insulin regimen and decide upon appropriate time for dialysis.
7 Check haematological state—evidence of DIC restore perfusion and oxygenation. Consider low dise heparin
8 Consider i.v. heparin infusion to prevent thrombosis
9 Use routine *antacids* to reduce incidence of acute gastric erosions

4.7 Tables

Table 4.73. Specific aspects of management of acute pancreatitis

1 Insert a Ryles tube, drain stomach. Use antacids routinely. No oral fluids
2 Use drugs for pain relief with care, respiratory depression is common. Preferable—continuous low dose infusion of opiate (subcut. or i.v.) 15-80 mg papaveretum/24 h. *Observe for respiratory depression*
3 Severe continuous pain, consider peritoneal lavage using a peritoneal dialysis catheter percutaneously or postoperatively via drain placed in the pancreatic bed. Use 500 ml isotonic dialysis solution ½-hourly continuous cycling
4 Observe for sepsis
   • repeated blood cultures
   • *do not use* prophylactic antibiotics
5 Sequential abdominal ultrasound to observe—changes in the pancreatic gland, early cyst or abscess formation, to exclude obstruction due to gallstones
6 *Supportive care*
   Maintenance of blood volume, metabolic balance and Se albumin.
   Maintenance of normal blood gases (ventilation may be necessary).
   Parenteral nutrition.
   Prevention of complications relating to stress and immobility.

Acute stress ulceration	— routine antacid therapy
Deep vein thrombosis	— prophylactic subcut heparin
Malnutrition and hypoalbuminaemia	— see above

7 *Surgery* indicated for refractory severe disease with no improvement on conservative management
   abscess
   cyst formation
   complicating perforation
   prolonged ileus with obstruction (generally >4/52 after onset of the disease)

4.0 Specific problems

4.7 Tables

Table 4.74. Summary of emergency treatment of poisoning

1 Check airway. Remove dentures, clear mouth of food or vomit (using a gauze swab to cover the index finger). Suck out bronchial secretions. Insert an airway
2 Nurse in coma position. Vomiting is common
3 Confirm the heart is beating, if not, intubate, ventilate and start cardiac massage
4 Assess adequacy of ventilation—give 100% oxygen via face mask. Manifest poor airway control and/or hypoventilation consider planned intubation (using a muscle relaxant if necessary) and artificial ventilation
5 Assess haemodynamic state. Treat
6 Take samples of
   • blood ⎫
   • stomach aspirate ⎬ for poisons analysis
   • urine ⎭
   • blood samples for   Astrup analysis
                         BU electrolytes
                         Hb PCV

   More tests may be required with certain suspected intoxication (e.g. X-ray of abdomen for lead poisoning)
7 Measure skin/core temperature—rewarm if necessary
8 Consider gastric lavage—consider any specific method of delaying absorption
9 Correct any acid base or metabolic abnormality. Treat if necessary any adverse intoxicant effect e.g. convulsions, cardiac dysrhythmias
10 Check if there is any specific antidote. Promote elimination if possible
11 Consider support for organ failure
12 Where treatment is in doubt consult the nearest poisons reference service (see appendix on p. 249)

Table 4.75. The use of forced alkaline diuresis in drug intoxication (in decreasing order of effective drug removal)

Salicylic acid
Probenecid
Acetyl salicylic acid
Phenylbutazone
Tolbutamide
Phenobarbitone
Nitrofurantoin
Cyclobarbitone

Table 4.76. Forced alkaline diuresis

Principle maintain urine flow at 250-500 ml/h
Maintain urine pH at 7.5-8.5.
1 Set up RAP. Catheterize
2 Check electrolytes, acid base balance and urine pH
3 *Do not* start until Se K >3.6 mmol/l, do not use if RAP >10 cm H_2O or there is a previous history of cardiac failure
4 Give normal saline or Haemaccel until RAP is >2 cm H_2O then commence:-
   • 500 ml 1/5 N saline + 50 mmol sodium bicarbonate
   • 500 ml N saline × potassium chloride 20-40 mmol (according to Se K)
   • Alternate hourly to 2 hourly
   • Adjust ratio of fluid mixtures in order to maintain urine pH at 7.5 or greater (may be necessary to use bicarbonate mixture alone)
5 Observe urine output and fluid balance. If RAP >6 cm H_2O and fluid retention occurring give burinex 1 mg i.v. *provided* Se K is >4.0, and slow down infusion rate until diuresis has occurred
6 Stop technique once serum salicylate in the asymptomatic range (see figure on p. 170) or barbiturate level below toxic range (see table on p. 24)

4.0 Specific problems

4.7 Tables

Table 4.77. Management of salicylate intoxication

1 Gastric lavage if ingestion <24 h. Give regular mist. mag. trisil. mixture via the Ryles tube

2 Check salicylate level, Astrup electrolytes, clotting factors. If salicylate level mild (see figure on p. 170) ensure a high fluid turnover rate 4 l/24 h and repeat salicylate level 2 h later

3 Salicylate level moderate to severe (see figure on p. 170) Insert RAP line measure biochemical state 2 hourly. Observe urine output, maintain careful fluid balance.

4 If pH <7.35 commence forced alkaline diuresis (see Table 4.76). Observe for complications including metabolic alkalosis → resp. depression.
   pH >7.35, establish a high fluid turnover rate 4-6 l/24 h alternating 1 l N saline with 1 l of 1/5 N saline
   Add potassium chloride approximately 120 mmol/24 h provided urine output maintained.
   Stop fluid load if RAP >6 cm H_2O
   Arterial pH monitoring is essential—alkalosis common initially (secondary to hyperventilation) which may slowly change to a metabolic and respiratory acidosis. $PaCO_2$ >5.0 kPa is an indication for intubation and ventilation. (During ventilation maintain $PaCO_2$ around 3.0 kPa).

5 Give vitamin K routinely

6 Check skin/core temperature if core temperature >40°C cool

7 BP SP <80 mmHg use dopamine infusion to maintain urine output

8 Renal failure—institute peritoneal dialysis immediately

9 Check salicylate blood level 2 hourly and *do not* cease careful biochemical monitoring until level <80 mg/100 ml on two consecutive occasions

Table 4.78. Management of digoxin intoxication

1 Induce vomiting with syrup of ipecacuanha (15-30 ml). Give activated charcoal 50-100 g for adults (25 g for children)
2 Treat hyperkalaemia with insulin and dextrose if Se K >6.5 mmol and exchange resin if Se K 5.5-6.5 mmol/l (see table on p. 185)
3 Treat dysrhythmia:
   - bradycardia pulse rate <50/min or <60/min with ventricular extrasystoles give atropine 300-600 μg in an adult, 10 μg/kg in a child
   - ventricular premature beats when frequent and close to the T wave give phenytoin sodium at a rate of 50 mg/min to a maximum dosage of 250 mg
   - if unsuccessful consider lignocaine 1-2 mg/kg i.v. followed by 1-3 mg/min as an infusion
   - A/V block, Se K >5.5 mmol/l, pulse rate <50/min unresponsive to atropine insert a pacing wire
     Pace at a rate which suppresses ventricular premature beats and twice the threshold for diastolic excitability
4 Immunological inactivation. In severe digoxin toxicity with cardiac deterioration inspite of the above measures consult local poisons reference service regarding use of sheep digoxin-specific antibody
5 Renal dialysis is not effective for digoxin removal. Commence peritoneal dialysis if Se K >6.0 mmol and renal failure present

Table 4.79. Management of organophosphorous poisoning

1 Complete rest; remove all clothing; wash skin thoroughly
2 Suck out secretions. Evidence of respiratory failure intubate and ventilate
3 Atropine give 2 mg i.m. or i.v. and repeat until full atropinization has occurred (dry skin, dry mouth, rapid pulse). Dose may be up to 1.0 g in the first 24 h
4 Pralidoxime (a cholinesterase reactivator) give 1.0 g i.v. and repeat upto two more doses if exposure within the last 24 h. (Pralidoxime available through the pharmacy from a local designated hospital)

4.0 Specific problems

4.7 Tables

Table 4.80. Management of paraquat poisoning

1 Treatment unnecessary where urine for paraquat is negative or the plasma level is below the line (see figure on p. 172)
2 Aspirate the stomach. Leave in stomach 200 ml of a 30% aqueous suspension of Fullers earth and 5 g of magnesium sulphate in 100 ml of water. Repeat 12 hours later
3 Organ failure support. Do not ventilate until PaO_2 <8 kPa (60 mmHg) avoid an FiO_2 of greater than 0.5.

4.8 References

Bayliss P. H. (1981) Disorders of antidiuretic hormone secretion. *Medicine*, **1**, 249.

Cohen R. D. (1978) Acute disorders of calcium metabolism. In *Medical Management of the Critically Ill Patient* (Ed. by G. C. Hanson & P. L. Wright), p. 198. Academic Press, London.

Done A. K. (1960) Salicylate intoxication: Significance of salicylate in blood in cases of acute ingestion. *Paediatrics*, **26**, 801.

Edelman I. S. & Liebman J. (1959) Anatomy of body weight electrolytes. *Am. J. Med.* **27**, 256.

Gronert G. A. (1980) Malignant hyperthermia. *Anaesthesiology*, **53**, 395.

Jennett B., Gleave J. & Wilson P. (1981) Brain death in three neurosurgical units. *Brit. Med. J.* **281**, 533.

Pallis C. (1982) ABC of brain stem death. Diagnosis of brain stem death I. *Brit. Med. J.* **285**, 1558.

Pallis C. (1982) ABC of brain stem death. Diagnosis of brain stem death II. *Brit. Med. J.* **285**, 1641.

Posner J. B. (1978) Coma and other states of consciousness. The differential diagnosis of brain death. *Ann. N.Y. Acad. Sci.* **315**, 215.

Prescott L. F., Park J., Sutherland G. R., Smith I. J. & Proudfoot A. F. (1976) Cysteamine, methionine and penicillamine in the treatment of paracetamol poisoning. *Lancet*, **ii**, 109.

Proudfoot A. T., Stewart M. S., Levitt T. & Widdop B. (1979) Paraquat poisoning: significance of plasma paraquat concentrations. *Lancet*, **ii**, 330.

Stone P. & Wright P. L. (1978) The management of poisoning. In *Medical Management of the Critically Ill Patient* (Ed. by G. C. Hanson & P. L. Wright), p. 611. Academic Press, London.

Working Party on behalf of the Health Departments of Great Britain and N. Ireland (1983) *Cadaveric organs for transplantation. A code of practice including the diagnosis of brain death.*

Wright P. L. (1978) Management of endocrine emergencies. In *Medical Management of the Critically Ill Patient* (Ed. by G. C. Hanson & P. L. Wright), p. 641. Academic Press, London.

4.0 Specific problems

Notes

Useful values (by H. E. R. Chew)

1 **Blood, 239**
   Biochemical values
   Endocrine indices
   Trace metals
   Haematological indices
   Coagulation

2 **Cerebrospinal fluid, 241**

3 **Renal function and urinary values, 241**

4 **Haemodynamic indices and derived values, 242**
   Normal pressures of right heart and pulmonary artery
   Body surface area
   Derived values

5 **Miscellaneous useful values, 243**
   Approximate allowances for net insensible loss
   Sweating
   Approximate volume of body fluid compartments
   Respiratory physiology

1 Blood

Biochemical values

Amylase (S or P)	70-300 μ/l
Aspartate aminotransferase (P)	6-42 μ/l
Bicarbonate (P)	22-32 mmol/l
Bilirubin	
(total) (S or P)	3-17 μmol/l
(direct) (S or P)	2-9 μmol/l
Calcium	2.10-2.70 mmol/l
Chloride	98-108 mmol/l
Creatinine	
Creatine (P)	5-120 μmol/l
Creatinine phosphokinase (P)	20-130 μ/l
Glucose (fasting) (fluoride) (P)	2.9-6.2 mmol/l
Lactate (special collection)	
arterial	0.3-0.8 mmol/l
venous	0.56-2.2 mmol l
LDH (S or P)	value depends upon technique
Magnesium (S or P)	0.7-1.1 mmol/l
Osmolality (S or P)	275-295 m osmol/kg
Phosphatase (alkaline) (S or P)	100-350 μ/l
Phosphate (inorganic) (P)	0.8-1.4 mmol/l
Potassium (P)	3.4-5.0 mmol/l
Proteins	
total (S)	63-78 g/l
albumin (S)	35-45 g/l
Sodium (P)	134-146 mmol/l
Urea (P)	3.0-8.0 mmol/l
Uric Acid (P)	
male	0.18-0.48 mmol/l
female	0.12-0.42 mmol/l

Endocrine indices

Cortisol (S or P)	
08.00-09.00 hours	300-800 nmol/l
16.00-17.00 hours	100-600 nmol/l
Growth hormone (fasting, resting) (S)	value depends upon technique
Thyroxine (S) T4	60-150 nmol/l
Triiodothyronine (S) T3	1.3-2.9 nmol/l
TSH (S)	1-5 m iu/l

Useful values

1 Blood

Trace metals

Copper (S or P)	11-23 μmol/l
Iron (S or P)	
male	14-31 μmol/l
female	11-29 μmol/l
Lead (HWB)	<2 μmol/l
Zinc (P)	12-20 μmol/l

Haematological indices

Red cell count	
male	5.5 ± 1.0 4.5-6.5×10^{12}/l
female	4.8 ± 1.0 3.8-5.8×10^{12}/l
Haemoglobin	
male	15.5 ± 2.5 g/dl
	13.0-18.0 g/dl
female	14.0 ± 2.5 g/dl
	13.5-16.5 g/dl
Haematocrit	
male	0.47 ± 0.07 0.40-0.54
female	0.42 ± 0.05 0.37-0.47
Mean corpuscular volume	85 ± 8.0 fl 77-93 fl
	(femtolitres)
Mean corpuscular haemoglobin (MCH)	29.5 ± 2.5 pg 27.0-32.0 pg
	(picograms)
MCH concentration MCHC	33 ± 2 g/dl 31-35 g/dl
Reticulocytes (0.2-2.0%)	10-100%
Leucocytes	7.5 ± 3.5 7.5-11.0×10^9/l
Differential leucocyte count	
neutrophils 40-75%	2.0-7.5×10^9/l
lymphocytes 20-45%	1.5-4.0×10^9/l
monocytes 2-10%	0.2-0.8×10^9/l
eosinophils 1-6%	0.04-0.4×10^9/l
basophils <1%	$<0.1\times10^9$/l
Platelets	150-$400\times10_9$/l
Serum iron	14-29 μmol/1
Total iron binding capacity	45-75 μmol/l
Serum B_{12}	160-925 ng/l
Serum folate 3-20 μg/l	3.20 μg/l
Transferrin	value depends upon technique

Useful values

Coagulation

Bleeding time	3 to 9 min (Simplate)
Whole blood clotting time	< 10 min
Kaolin cephalin time	35-45 sec
(partial thromboplastin time)	
Prothrombin time	10-14 sec
Thrombin time	Consult your laboratory
Fibrinogen level	165-485 mg/100 ml
Fibrinogen titre	> 1/64
Fibrin degradation products	value depends upon technique

2 Cerebrospinal fluid

Protein 0.13-0.45 g/l
Glucose 2.7-4.2 mmol/l (approx 60% of blood level)

3 Renal function and urinary values

GFR	100-150 ml/min 1.73 m^2 (non-pregnant adults)
Max. urinary conc.	> 800 mosmol/kg
pH	4.5-8.0
SG	1010-1025
Volume	800-2000 ml/24 h
Sodium	variable
Calcium	2.5-7.5 mmol/24 h
Chloride	100-250 mmol/24 h
Magnesium	2.0-10.0 mmol/24 h
Potassium	35-90 mmol/24 h
Creatinine	8.0-18.0 mmol/24 h
Urea	167-500 mmol/24 h
Vanillylmandelic acid (VMA)	up to 45 μmol/24 h
Adrenaline	< 109 mmol/24 h
Nor-adrenaline	< 591 mmol/24 h
Creatinine clearance	95-135 ml/min (non-pregnant adults)

4   Haemodynamic indices and derived values

Normal pressures of right heart and pulmonary artery

Site	Pressure (mmHg)
Right atrium	
Mean	-1-$+7$
Right ventricle	
Systolic	15-25
Diastolic	0-8
Pulmonary artery	
Systolic	15-25
Diastolic	8-15
Mean	10-20
Pulmonary capillary wedge	
Mean	6-15

Mean level at which pulmonary oedema is likely in relation
to serum albumin

Cardiac output (CO)	$0.57 \times$ serum albumen g/l
Cardiac index	4.0-8.0 l/min
	cardiac output
	body surface area

$$= 3.0 \pm 0.5 \text{ l/min/m}^2$$

Body surface area

Weight (kg)	Surface area (m²)
30	1.05
40	1.30
50	1.50
60	1.65
70	1.75
80	1.85
90	1.95
100	2.05

Useful values

5 Miscellaneous useful values

Derived values

$$LVSWI = \frac{1.36 \times (MAP - PCWP) \times SVI}{100}$$
$$= 45 - 60 \text{ gm} - M/M^2/\text{beat}$$

$$MAP = DP + \frac{1}{3}(SP - DP)$$

$$PVR = \frac{PAP - PCWP}{CO} \times 80 = 50 - 150 \text{ Dyne/sec/cm}^{-5}$$

$$SV = \frac{CO}{HR} = 60 - 100 \text{ ml/beat}$$

$$SVI = \frac{CO \times 1000 \text{ ml/L}}{BSA \times HR} = 40 \pm 7 \text{ ml/beat/M}^2$$

$$SVR = \frac{MAP - RAP}{CO} \times 80 = 800 - 1200 \text{ Dyne/sec/cm}^{-5}$$

5 Miscellaneous useful values

Approximate allowances for net insensible loss

Average daily core temperature (°C)	Net insensible loss (ml)
Normal	350
37.2	400
37.8	500
38.3	600
38.9	700
39.4	900

Sweating

Add quantity to insensible loss.
Sweating generally produces a fall in body temperature.
Pyrexia often produced by a failure to sweat.
Mild—(involving axilla and pubic region)
Moderate—the above plus scalp and face
Severe—involving the whole of the body

Mild intermittent	300 ml/day
Moderate intermittent	600 ml/day
Severe intermittent	1000 ml/day

Useful values

5 Miscellaneous useful values

Continuous sweating 2-15 l/day
If ventilated or breathing humidified gases allow half the calculated
quantities

Approximate volume of body fluid compartments

Body weight (kg)	40	50	60	70	80
ICF (L)	16	20	24	28	32
ECF (L) (including plasma)	8	10	12	14	16
Plasma (L)	1.7	2.1	2.5	3.0	3.5
Blood (L)	2.8	3.5	4.2	5.0	5.8

In females and obese males reduce ICF volume by 10%

Respiratory physiology

Tracheal dimensions	Length of trachea (cm)	Sagittal diam. of trachea (cm)	Coronal diam. of trachea (cm)
Neonate	4	0.5	0.6
6-8 years	5.5	1.0	1.1
14-16 years	7	1.0	1.3
Adult	11-12	1.6-2.0	1.4

From Gothard J. W. W. & Branthwaite M. A. (1982) *Anaesthesia for Thoracic Surgery*. Blackwell Scientific Publications, Oxford.

Blood

Arterial
  pH   7.36-7.44
  PaO_2 11.3-13.3 kPa (85-100 mmHg)
  $PaCO_2$ 4.8-5.9 kPa (36-44 mmHg)
  O_2 content   8.9-9.4 mmol/l (20-21 vol %)
  CO_2 content   21.6-22.5 mmol/l (48-50 vol %)

Useful values

5   Miscellaneous useful values

Gases

Inspired air
  Oxygen 20.93%
  P_IO_2 19.9 kPa (149 mmHg)
  CO_2 0.03%
Expired air
  O_2 16-17%
  P_EO_2 15-16 kPa (113-121 mmHg)
  CO_2 3-4%
  P_ECO_2 2.8-3.7 kPa (21-28 mmHg)

Ventilation perfusion

Alveolar-arterial oxygen gradient	
breathing air	0.7-2.7 kPa (5-20 mmHg)
breathing 100% oxygen	3.3-8.6 kPa (25-65 mmHg)
Right to left physiological shunt	3% of cardiac output
Anatomical dead space	2 ml/kg body weight

Approximate lung volumes

Tidal volume	7 ml/kg
Total lung capacity	6.0 l
Vital capacity	2.5 l/m²BSA (males)
	2.0 l/m²BSA (females)
or	65-75 ml/kg.

Lung mechanics

Peak expiratory flow	450-700 l/min (males)
	300-500 l/min (females)
FEV_1	70-83% of vital capacity

Airways resistance

Conscious	0.6-3.2 cm H_2O/l/sec
Sedated paralysed and ventilated (volumes E-T tube and catheter mount)	approx. 10-15 cm H_2O/l/sec
Effective dynamic compliance i.e. total compliance in a ventilated sedated patient	40-50 ml/cm H_2O

Appendices

1 Poisons reference services, 249

2 List of abbreviations, 249

Appendices

1 Poisons reference services / 2 Abbreviations

1 Poisons reference services

Belfast	0232 30503
Cardiff	0222 492233
Dublin	0001 745588
Edinburgh	031 229 2477
Leeds	0532 32799
London	01 407 7600
Manchester	061 740 2254
Newcastle	0632 25131

2 List of abbreviations

ACTH	Adrenocorticol stimulating hormone
ADH	Antidiuretic hormone
AF	Atrial fibrillation
ARDS	Adult respiratory distress syndrome
ARF	Acute renal failure
A-V	Atrioventricular
AVP	Arginine vasopressin
BG	Blood glucose
BP	Blood pressure
BSA	Body surface area
BU	Blood urea
BUN	Blood urea nitrogen
BW	Body weight
Ca	Calcium
CAT	Computerized axial tomography
CCF	Congestive cardiac failure
CDI	Cranial diabetes insipidus
CHO	Carbohydrate
CI	Cardiac index
CL	Chloride
CNS	Central nervous system
CO	Cardiac output
CO_2	Carbon dioxide
COP	Colloid osmotic pressure
CPAP	Continuous positive airway pressure
CPPV	Continuous positive pressure ventilation
CRAP	Continuous raised airway pressure
CRF	Chronic renal failure
CSF	Cerebrospinal fluid
CVA	Cerebrovascular accident
CXR	Chest X-ray

Appendices

2 Abbreviations

d.c.	Direct current
DI	Diabetes insipidus
DIC	Disseminated intravascular coagulation
DKA	Diabetic ketoacidosis
DM	Diabetes mellitus
DP	Diastolic pressure
DPG	Diphosphoglycerate
ECM	External cardiac massage
E-T	Endotracheal
ETT	Endotracheal tube
FEV_1	Forced expiratory volume over 1 second
FFP	Fresh frozen plasma
FHF	Fulminant hepatic failure
F_iO_2	Inspired oxygen percentage
FVC	Forced vital capacity
GI	Gastro-intestinal
GU	Genito-urinary
H	Hydrogen
Hb	Haemoglobin
HBO	Hyperbaric oxygen
HCO_3	Bicarbonate
Hct	Haematocrit
HFMV	High frequency mechanical ventilation
HR	Heart rate
HWB	Heparin whole blood
IADH	Inappropriate release of antidiuretic hormone
ICP	Intracranial pressure
IHD	Ischaemic heart disease
i.m.	Intramuscular
IMV	Intermittent mandatory ventilation
IPPV	Intermittent positive pressure ventilation
ITU	Intensive Therapy Unit
i.v.	Intravenous
IVP	Intravenous pyelography
K	Potassium
K_2HPO_4	Dipotassium hydrogen phosphate
KPTT	Kaolin partial thromboplastin time
LAP	Left atrial pressure
LAT	Lateral
LDH	Lactic dehydrogenase
LH	Left hand
LP	Lumbar puncture
LV	Left ventricular or left ventricle
LVF	Left ventricular failure
LVFP	Left ventricular filling pressure

Appendices

2 Abbreviations

LVSWI	Left ventricular stroke work index
MAP	Mean arterial pressure
Mg	Magnesium
MU	Mega unit
Na	Sodium
NDI	Nephrogenic diabetes insipidus
NKA	Non-ketotic hyperglycaemia
OxyHb	Oxyhaemoglobin
P	Plasma
P_{50}	Pressure of oxygen in the arterial blood at 50 percent saturation haemoglobin
PA	Postero-anterior
$PaCO_2$	Arterial carbon dioxide pressure
PaO_2	Arterial oxygen pressure
PCV	Packed cell volume
PAP	Pulmonary artery pressure
PCWP	Pulmonary capillary wedge pressure
PEEP	Positive end expiratory pressure
pKa	Dissociation constant
PPF	Plasma protein fraction
P/r	Per rectum
P-T	Prothrombin time
PVR	Pulmonary vascular resistance
RAD	Right axis deviation
RAP	Right atrial pressure
RBC	Red blood cells
RH	Right hand
RHF	Right heart failure
RTA	Road traffic accident
RVH	Right ventricular hypertrophy
s.c.	Subcutaneous
SP	Systolic pressure
SV	Stroke volume
SVI	Stroke volume index
SVR	Systemic vascular resistance
SVT	Supraventricular tachycardia
T_3	Triiodothyronine
T_4	Thyroxine
TBW	Total body water
t.i.d.	Three times a day
TSH	Thyroid stimulating hormone
TSS	Toxin shock syndrome
U & E	Urea and electrolytes
U/P	Urine/plasma
VC	Vital capacity

Appendices

2 Abbreviations

VF	Ventricular fibrillation
VSD	Ventricular septal defect
VT	Ventricular tachycardia
W	Weight
WBC	White blood cell count
WPW	Wolff-Parkinson-White

Index

Abdominal injury 100-101, 121
Acid-base disorders 151-4
  Metabolic classification 190
  Respiratory classification 190
Acidosis, metabolic
  and anion gap 152
  causes 191
  consequences of 190-1
  lactic acidosis 153
    and diabetes mellitus 208
    classification 192
    conditions predisposing
      to 193
    treatment 194
Acute toxic shock syndrome
  (ATS) 110
Addisonian crisis *see* adrenal
  gland
Adrenal gland
  Acute hypercortisolism 158-9
    treatment 214
  Addisonian crisis 158
    manifestations 213
    treatment 214
  Phaeochromocytoma
    treatment 215-6
Adult respiratory distress
  syndrome (ARDS) 44-5
Alkalosis, metabolic 153-4
  and arginine monohydro-
    chloride 154, 196
  factors, mechanisms and
    treatment 195-6
Aminophylline
  dosage 83
Amiodarone
  in dysrhythmias 73, 76
Anaesthetic, local
  for chest injury 52, 53
Antacids
  and renal failure 66
Antibiotics
  and fat embolism 46
  and hepatic failure 58
  and meningitis 219

  and near drowning 46
  and pancreatitis 229
  and pneumonia 113
  and pulmonary aspiration 48
  and respiratory failure 41
  and shock and infection
    108, 128
  and ulcerative colitis 225
Anticonvulsants
  blood levels, toxic and thera-
    peutic 220
  in status epilepticus 220
Arginine monohydrochloride
  and metabolic alkalosis 154
    196
Aspiration syndrome 47-8
Asthma 49-50
Atrial fibrillation
  treatment of 36
Atropine
  in dysrhythmias 76
  in organophosphorous
    poisoning 233
  in polyneuritis 221

β Blockers
  and polyneuropathy 221
  Practolol
    in dysrhythmias 70
    in phaeochromocytoma
      216
  Propranolol
    in dysrhythmias 70
    in phaeochromocytoma
      216
  treatment of poisoning 168
Benzodiazepines 12
  classification of 23
Bicarbonate, sodium
  in forced alkaline diuresis
    231
  in lactic acidosis 194
  in metabolic acidosis 192
  in shock 117
  in shock and sepsis 105-6

Index

in the hyperosmolar syndrome 205, 207
Bradycardia
  cardiac pacing and 37
  in overdose 166
Brain stem death 162-3
Bretylium
  in dysrhythmias 76
Bronchodilators
  in asthma 49, 50, 83
  in respiratory failure 41

Calcium, disorders in 148-50
  hypercalcaemia 149-50
    causes 187
    treatment 187-8
  hypocalcaemia 148-9
    causes 186
    treatment 186
Cardiac
  arrest 31
    definition 31
    diagnosis 31
    treatment 31, 32, 67, 68
  arrhythmias 34
    atrial response to carotid sinus massage 74
    bradycardias 37
    causes 69
    drug treatment and 70-6
    fibrillation, ventricular 31
    in overdose 165
    supraventricular 35, 36
    ventricular 36, 37, 76
  arrhythmias, treatment
    atrial fibrillation 75
    atrial tachycardia 74
    junctional tachycardia 75
    nodal tachycardia 74
    supraventricular tachycardia 35
    WPW syndrome 74
  asystole
    causes 32
    treatment 32

depression in shock and sepsis 106, 107
failure 38
  drugs and 77, 78, 79
  treatment 38
Carotid sinus massage
  artrial dysrhythmias, response to 74
CAT scan
  and electrical and lightning injuries 123
  and head injury 98, 119
Cerebrospinal fluid
  in acute polyneuropathy 161
  in meningitis 160
Cholinergic crisis see myasthenia gravis
Cobalt edetate
  in poisoning 165-7
Coma
  hepatic 58
Continuous raised airway pressure (CRAP) 53, 54
Crohn's disease see inflammatory bowel disease
Cysteine and methionine
  in paracetamol poisoning 168,
  in poisoning 167

DC shock
  in cardiac arrest 32
Dexamethasone
  and head injury 119
Dextran 70   96
  and shock 116
Diabetes insipidus 217
  cranial 217
    treatment 218
  nephrogenic 217
    treatment 218
Diabetes mellitus see hyperosmolar syndrome related to diabetes mellitus

Index

Dialysis *see* renal dialysis
Digoxin/Digitalis
  and cardiac failure 77
  factors altering efficacy 75
  in dysrhythmias 73
  in shock 117
  poisoning and 169-70
    management 233
Disopyramide
  in dysrhythmias 71, 76
Disseminated intravascular
    coagulation (DIC)
  diagnosis 128
  in shock and sepsis 108
  treatment in shock and
    sepsis 129
Diuretics
  and cardiac failure 77
Dopamine hydrochloride
  in cardiac failure 77
  in poisoning 165
  in shock and sepsis 106, 127
Dobutamine
  in cardiac failure 78
  in poisoning 165
  in shock and sepsis 106, 127
Doxapram
  in respiratory failure 41
Drowning—near 46-7
Drug
  blood levels, toxic and thera-
    peutic 24, 25, 26
  hepatic failure and 22
  interactions 20
  metabolism 12
    of benzodiazepines 23
  renal failure and 20

Edrophonium test
  in myasthenia gravis 222
Electrical and lightning injury
    101-2
  complications 121-2
  management 122-4
Embolectomy
  for pulmonary embolism 48
Embolism
  pulmonary 48
Encephalopathy
  hepatic grading 86
Endocrine crisis 158-60
  related to
    the adrenal gland 158-9
    the pituitary and hypo-
      thalamus 159-60
    the thyroid gland 158
Epilepsy
  status 161
    anticonvulsant blood levels
      220
    factors precipitating 219
    treatment 220-1

Fat embolism 45
Fluid
  and overload 95
    causes 114
  challenge and RAP 105
  in shock and sepsis 104-5
  ratios to give in severe
    haemorrhage 118
  types for volume replace-
    ment 95-6

Gastro-intestinal emergencies
    163-4
  acute pancreatitis 164
  haemorrhage 163
  inflammatory bowel disease
    163-4
Guillain-Barré syndrome *see*
    polyneuropathy

Haemoperfusion
  in poisoning 167
Haemorrhage
  and DIC 128
  and shock management 96-8
  causes 114
  gastro-intestinal 163

Index

management 223-4
gastro-intestinal and hepatic
    failure 56-7
severity 115
source of 96
summary of treatment 116-7
volume loss in injury 118
Haemaccel 96
    and shock 116
Heat stroke *see* hyperthermia
H_2 antagonists
    and renal failure 64
Head injury
    management 119
    observations 99
Heparin
    and pulmonary embolism 48
    in DIC 129
Hepatic failure
    and poisoning 167, 168
    clinical features 55, 56
    definition 55
    drugs and 22
    encephalopathy grading 86
    factors precipitating 85
    fulminant (FHF) 55
        causes 85
    treatment 55-9
Hydralazine
    in cardiac failure 78
    in hypertension 80
Hydrocortisone
    and Addisonian crisis 214
    and asthma 49
    and fat embolism syndrome
        46
    and hypercortisolism 207
    and hypopituitary coma 217
    and myxoedema coma 211
    and near drowning 46
    and pulmonary aspiration 47
    and thyroid crisis 213
    and ulcerative colitis 225
Hypercortisolism *see* adrenal
    gland

Hyperglycaemia
    and the hyperosmolar syn-
        drome
        causes 206
        treatment 156
            related to diabetes
                mellitus 156-7, 207
            unrelated to diabetes
                mellitus 155-6, 205
    diagnosis 194
Hyperkalaemia 146-7
    causes 184
    ECG and 147
    treatment 148, 185
Hypernatraemia 145
    complications 204
    diagnosis 156, 200
    management 203-4
Hyperosmolar syndromes
        (including diabetes
        mellitus) 155-7
    associated with diabetes
        mellitus 156-7
    factors producing 202
    unrelated to diabetes
        mellitus 155-6
Hyperosmolar syndrome re-
        lated to diabetes
        mellitus 156-7
    diabetic ketoacidosis 156-7
        diagnosis 206
        management 207-8
    non-ketotic hyperglycaemia
        157
        management 208-9
Hyperosmolar syndrome un-
        related to diabetes
        mellitus 155-6
    management 155-6, 203-4,
        205
Hypertension
    acute 39
    drugs and rapid reduction 80
    procedure for reduction 81
Hyperthermia

Index

heat stroke 141-2
  clinical features 142
  drugs predisposing to 173
  treatment 173-4
  hyperpyrexia, malignant 142-3
Hypokalaemia 145-6
  causes 182
  ECG and 146
  treatment 176
Hyponatraemia
  diagnosis 201
  diagnosis and treatment 176-7
  in myxoedema coma 211
Hypothermia
  complications 141
  features 139-40
  treatment 140-1

Infection
  acute toxic shock syndrome 110
  anaerobic 109
  pneumonia 113, 131, 132, 133
  tetanus 110-12, 130, 131
Inflammatory bowel disease
  diagnosis and management 225
    Crohn's disease 164
    treatment 226
    ulcerative colitis 163-4
    treatment 225
Injuries
  chest 50-3
    classification 84
    physiological consequences of 52
Inotropes
  and cardiac failure 77, 78
  and pulmonary embolism 48
  in poisoning 165
  in shock and sepsis 106, 127
Isosorbide dinitrate

in cardiac failure 79
Intensive therapy unit
  definition 7
  function of 7
  indications for admission to 7
  monitoring in 7
  treatment priorities in 8
Isoprenaline hydrochloride
  in cardiac failure 78

Labetolol
  in hypertension 80
Lactic acidosis
  see acidosis metabolic
Lavage
  bronchial in asthma 50
  gastric in overdose 166
Lignocaine
  in dysrhythmias 71, 76
Liver
  failure see hepatic failure

Magnesium deficiency 150
  causes for 188
  treatment 189
Mannitol
  in shock 117, 119
Meningitis 160
  causes 218
  diagnosis 160
  treatment 219
Metabolic
  acid-base disorders 152-4
    primary metabolic acidosis 152-3
    primary metabolic alkalosis 153-4
Metabolic disorders 153-7
  disorders in acid-base balance 151-4
  disorders in calcium and magnesium balance 148-50
  disorders in phosphate

257

Index

balance 151
disorders in porphyrin metabolism 154
disorders in potassium balance 145-8
disorders in uric acid metabolism 154
disorders in water and sodium balance 143-5
hyperosmolar states (incl. diabetes mellitus) 155-7
response to stress 143
Methionine *see* cysteine
Mexilitine
in dysrhythmias 71, 76
Monitoring
systems
invasive 18-19
non-invasive 14-17
Myasthenia gravis 162
cholinergic crisis 162
treatment 223
myasthenic crisis 162
treatment 222
Myxoedema *see* thyroid gland

Naloxone hydrochloride
in poisoning 166
Nitroprusside
in cardiac failure 79
in hypertension 80
Neostigmine methyl sulphate
in myasthenia gravis 222-3
Nervous system
disorders of 160-1
brain stem death 162-3
meningitis 160
myasthenia gravis 162
polyneuropathies 161-2
status epilepticus 161
Noradrenaline
and pulmonary embolism 48

Opiates and cardiac failure 77
Organ failure
cardiac 31
hepatic 55
renal 60
respiratory 40
Organophosphorus poisoning 170-1
treatment 233
Osmolality
diagnosis of intracellular and extracellular volume changes 200
diagnosis of oliguria 86
Overdose *see* poisoning
Oxygen
therapy 41
toxicity 45
Oxyhaemoglobin dissociation curve
and metabolic acidosis 191
and metabolic alkalosis 153
P_{50} *see also* oxyhaemoglobin dissociation curve
factors which may lower 115
Pancreatitis 164
complications 227
indications for admission to ITU 226
treatment 228, 229
Paracetamol
blood levels and liver damage 169
treatment of poisoning 168-9
Paraquat poisoning 171
blood levels and prognosis 172
management 234
products of 171
Phaeochromocytoma *see* adrenal gland
Phenoxybenzamine
and phaeochromocytoma 216
Phentolamine
and phaeochromocytoma 215, 216

Index

Phenytoin
  in dysrhythmias 72, 76
Phosphate
  deficiency 151
  treatment 189
Pituitary gland and hypo-
        thalamus 159-60
  diabetes insipidus 160
    causes 217
    treatment 218
  hypopituitary coma 159-60
    manifestations 216-7
    treatment 217
Pneumonia 113
  diagnosis of infection type
        132
  organisms involved 131
Poisoning 164-72
  reference services 249
  treatment, antidotes in 166-7
  treatment, forced diuresis
        167, 231
  treatment, general 165-7,
        230
  treatment, particular
        aspects 167
  treatment, specific manage-
        ment 168-72
Polyneuropathy acute 161-2
  treatment 221-2
Porphyria acute 154-5
  and porphyrin blood level
        changes 197
  drugs and factors precipitat-
        ing 198
  treatment 199
Porphyrin
  disorders in metabolism
        154-5
  normal levels 197
Potassium see also hypo-
        kalaemia, hyperkalaemia
  compartmental shifts 181
  depletion 145-6, 182-3
  disorders in balance 145-8

  excess 146-8, 184, 185
Potassium iodide
  in thyroid crisis 213
PPF 96
  and shock 116, 120
Pralidoxime
  in organophosphorous
        poisoning 233
Prednisolone
  in asthmá 49
  in shock and sepsis 106
  in ulcerative colitis 225
Procainamide
  in dysrhythmias 72, 76
Pyridostigmine bromide
  in myasthenia gravis 222,
        223

Receptors α and β 215
Renal dialysis 64-5
  in poisoning 167
  in the hyperosmolar syn-
        drome 203, 204, 208
Renal failure
  and haemorrhage 97
  and hepatic failure 59
  and poisoning 167, 232
  complications 63-4
  definition 60
  diagnosis 86
  dialysis 64-5
  drugs and 20, 21, 22
  factors precipitating 87-9
  treatment
    acute renal failure 63-6
    post-renal 61-2
    pre-renal 61
Respiratory failure
  causes 40, 81-2
  definition 40
  physiotherapy in 83
  treatment 41-4
Right atrial pressure and fluid
        challenge 105

Index

Salbutamol
  dosage 83
Salicylate intoxication 169
  blood levels and severity 170
  management 232
Sengstaken — Blakemore tube
  and oesophageal bleeding
    57
Shock 93-134
  definition 95
  due to changes in blood
    volume 95-8
  due to sepsis 102-13
  pathophysiology 95
Shock and sepsis
  and myocardial deppression
    107
  and surgery 108-9
  antibiotics and 128
  diagnosis 124
  DIC and 108, 128, 129
  inotropes and 127
  metabolic control 105-6
  monitoring and 126-7
  pathophysiology 102
    pre-, per- and postopera-
      tive preparation 129-30
  treatment, sequence 125
    summary 125-6
  unusual types
    acute toxic shock
      syndrome 110
    anaerobic 109
Sick sinus syndrome
  treatment of 36
Sodium see also hypo-
    natraemia, hyper-
    natraemia
  disorders in balance 114-5
  excess (hypernatraemia) 145
  serum concentration
    abnormalities in
      145, 175
  shift (the sick cell) 145, 175
  total body depletion 144, 175

  quantity lost, 180
  treatment 179
Spinal injury
  management 100, 120
Streptokinase
  and pulmonary embolism 48
Stress
  and metabolic response 143

T_3 T_4
  in myxoedema coma 211
Tachycardia
  supraventricular 35
    paroxysmal 35, 36, 74
  torsade de pointes
    treatment 76
  ventricular
    treatment 36, 37, 76
Temperature disorders 139-43
  hyperpyrexia, malignant
    142-3
  hyperthermia 141-3
  hypothermia 139-41
Tetanus
  diagnosis 110-11
  treatment 111-2
Thyroid gland
  myxoedema coma 158
    manifestations 210
    precipitating factors 209
    treatment 210-11
  thyroid crisis 158
    manifestations 212
    treatment 212-13
Tocainide
  in dysrhythmias 71, 76
Trauma see also injury and
    specific injuries
  particular aspects of 98-102
  types
    abdominal injury 100-1
    burns 101
    electrical and lightning
      101-2
    head injuries 100-2

of the genito-urinary tract
101
spinal injuries 100
Treatment
efficacy 13
interactions 10
enzyme induction 10
in excretory mechanisms
11
oral 10
plasma and receptor bind-
ing sites 11
site 11
pharmacology 9
principles of 8
priorities 8
Tricyclic antidepressants
treatment of poisoning 168

Ulcerative colitis *see* inflammatory bowel disease
Uric acid
excess 154

Vasodilators, peripheral
hydralazine 78, 90
isosorbide dinitrate 79
nitroprusside 79, 80

Vasopressin
in variceal haemorrhage 57
Ventilation
and calculation of F_iO_2 43
in head injury 123
in shock and sepsis 103
intermittent mandatory 44,
53
mechanical 42, 53
sedation for 42
ventilatory weaning 42
Ventricular fibrillation
causes 33
treatment 33
Verapamil
in dysrhythmias 70

Water
depletion 144, 174-5
diagnosis 200
disorders in 143-5
intoxication 144-5
diagnosis 200
total body in relation to age
and sex 205
Wolff-Parkinson-White
syndrome
treatment of 36